AYNI BOOKS

"Ayni" is a Quechua word meaning "reciprocity" – sharing, giving and receiving – whatever you give out comes back to you. To be in Ayni is to be in balance, harmony and right relationship with oneself and nature, of which we are all an intrinsic part. Complementary and Alternative approaches to health and well-being essentially follow a holistic model, within which one is given support and encouragement to move towards a state of balance, true health and wholeness, ultimately leading to the awareness of one's unique place in the Universal jigsaw of life – Ayni, in fact.

About the Author

Machel Shull is the author of the international bestselling book, *Middle Age Beauty*, an inspirational self-help book for women. Her background and study includes seven years of meditation with Michiko Jane Rolek, the great-granddaughter of the first Zen Master in America, Sokei-an Sasaki. *Live Love Soul: A Soul's Guide to Happy* is her second non-fiction book. Machel lives in Cardiff-by-the-Sea, California with her husband, teenage son, two cats and a red Doberman. Her coffee nickname is "Mimi." She is currently working on her third book, *Happy Soul*. Her background includes writing a newspaper column for five years in Rancho Santa Fe, plus writing travel, health and fashion features for magazines in Southern California. Machel was also featured on the Mind Body Green website in 2014. Besides writing and spending time with her family, Machel loves yoga, reading and eating sushi with her girlfriends.

*If you are looking for a life coach, Michiko Jane Rolek, my mentor and teacher, can be contacted through her website at funzenbakery.com or Twitter page. My work with her as my teacher has been instrumental in me discovering my life path and living my dreams.

*Research and quotes listed in *Live Love Soul: A Soul's Guide to Happy* are given credit to rightful sources.

Lilacs

Lilacs represent the beginning of spring and are known as a designator that winter is over. Just like our soul hibernates and rejuvenates itself over the years, lilacs bloom again in the spring. Their lavender and purple petals reach up to the sun and find the light again when winter has begun to fade. A new beginning is always possible. Let the lilacs be a reminder to find our own bloom and rediscover our beauty of life.

275

Live Love Soul

A Soul's Guide to *Happy*

Machel Shull

AYNI BOOKS

Winchester, UK
Washington, USA

First published by Ayni Books, 2015
Ayni Books is an imprint of John Hunt Publishing Ltd., Laurel House, Station Approach,
Alresford, Hants, SO24 9JH, UK
office1@jhpbooks.net
www.johnhuntpublishing.com
www.ayni-books.com

For distributor details and how to order please visit the 'Ordering' section on our website.

Text copyright: Machel Shull 2014

ISBN: 978 1 78279 284 0
Library of Congress Control Number: 2014958259

A CIP catalogue record for this book is available from the British Library.

Design: Stuart Davies

Printed and bound in the USA by Edwards Brothers Malloy

We operate a distinctive and ethical publishing philosophy in all
areas of our business, from our global network of authors to
production and worldwide distribution.

LIVE LOVE SOUL

Machel's beautiful, honest and easy to use guide shows you exact steps to infuse happiness into your daily life. Machel proves you don't have to go to India and sit on a mountaintop somewhere to find your bliss. You can find it right here, right now. Her book is an invaluable resource for women ready to reclaim their happy! **Rosemond Perdue Cranner** *A former entertainment executive, Rosemond has produced web content for The Discovery Channel, HGTV, MTV and Animal Planet, and was the creator of Lifetime Television's first scripted web series, "Mommy Madness." She is also the Founder/Blogger: roundandroundrosie.com ~A Blog about your amazing life after divorce*

Machel has written a very liberating book which acts as a roadmap for tapping into the wellspring of peace, joy and happiness. Though written in a light-hearted manner, this book has the power to totally transform your life.
Mary Elizabeth Coen, *International Bestselling Irish Author of* Love and the Goddess

Some say, "Don't judge a book by its cover." With Machel, what you'll find is that what's soul deep on the inside is just as beautiful as the cover. Read on and see for yourself. And most importantly, let Machel inspire you to reach inward to be the superhero of your own story.
Michiko Jane Rolek, *Author, Teacher, Lecturer and Life Coach. She was born into a famous Zen lineage*

Whether you need to find a new direction for your life, or reconnect with yourself, this book will give you the tools. A must-read for anyone on the path of soul discovery.

Monica Cafferky, *British Journalist and Author*

Live Love Soul

A Soul's Guide to *Happy*

CONTENTS

Acknowledgements   xii

Foreword   1

Dear Readers   4

Introduction   8

Part One — Live   **15**

Chapter 1. Oh, the Small Joys   17

Chapter 2. This Too Shall Pass   21

Chapter 3. Don't Leave Home without These Three Things   27

Chapter 4. Bloom Where You Are Planted on
Independence Day   37

Chapter 5. Interview — with Legendary Free-Range
Snowboarder, Jeremy Jones   43

Chapter 6. Have a Bucket List   49

Chapter 7. How to Stay Motivated   55

Chapter 8. Breaking through the Walls   61

Chapter 9. Be Flexible. Life Can Change on a Dime   69

Chapter 10. Why *Trying* Is Something You Should Do   75

Chapter 11. The Ladder of Life — Reach Up and Grab On   83

Chapter 12. Interview — with Dr Jason Karp on the
Benefits of Exercise and Running   91

Part Two — Love   **97**

Chapter 13. Non Judgment. Melt Your Heart from
Judging by Inserting These Two Words   99

Chapter 14. Take 'Mini-Me' Breaks and Discover the
Gift of Solitude   105

Chapter 15. Extend the White Rose of Love and What
Would *Harvey* Do?   111

Chapter 16. Cultivate More Self-Love   117

Chapter 17. Interview—with #1 Bestselling Author from
    Ireland, Mary Elizabeth Coen   123
Chapter 18. Move On or Move Out If Those You Love Feed
    Negativity and Self-Doubt   131
Chapter 19. The Three S's for Helping You Find More
    Love and Happiness   137
Chapter 20. One More Day Can Make the Difference. Keep
    Looking toward the Heavenly Stars   145
Chapter 21. Interview—with Matchmaker Elle France on
    Why Matters of the Heart…Matter   151
Chapter 22. Empathy and Why We Need More of It   159

Part Three—Soul   **163**
Chapter 23. Have a Little *Soul*   165
Chapter 24. The Power of Sharing and Honoring Each
    Other's Stories   169
Chapter 25. Interview—with Author and Zen Life Coach,
    Michiko Jane Rolek   177
Chapter 26. Why Believing in Something Matters   185
Chapter 27. Designing the Book Cover of Your Life   191
Chapter 28. Non Attachment and Finding a Balance   201
Chapter 29. Why Appearance Matters to Your Soul   205
Chapter 30. Interview—with Rock Star Violinist,
    Lindsey Stirling   213
Chapter 31. Grief and Pain—How Do We Carry On?   221
Chapter 32. Quiet Time for the Soul—Even If It Lands
    On Your Birthday   227
Chapter 33. Interview—with Dr Doris Lee McCoy on the
    Search for Happiness   233
Chapter 34. Get Happy by Loving Yourself. You Are a
    Rock Star   239
Chapter 35. The Soul Kit. Three Little Things You Need
    for a Rainy Day   243
Chapter 36. Tidy the Soul   251

Chapter 37. The Safety Net for the Soul   259
Chapter 38. Interview—with You, Dear Reader. Unlock
    Your Goals and Dreams   267
Chapter 39. Epilogue   273

About the Author   275

For, my parents, William and Micky Penn

And

My husband, Robin Shull and my son, Jackson Tuck

Acknowledgements

I would like to acknowledge Tess Hightower and Michiko Jane Rolek for teaching me during a transitional time to follow my heart and develop my passion. This book is essentially that story, plus interviews from extraordinary individuals that share their secrets on how they keep pursuing their dreams.

Also, thank you to my mother, Micky Kay Penn for always being my first reader. I am so blessed to have you as my mom. Thank you also to my dad for always encouraging me to believe in myself and to follow my dreams. Your words of wisdom have guided and inspired me over the years. Thank you to Ayni Books for giving this book an opportunity to find wings for its readers.

Foreword

To find oneself, at 25, working as a model and actress in Hollywood would seem like the perfect dream to any young woman. Surely it must take something a lot bigger to lure a girl away from the hope of achieving international fame and fortune? Grace Kelly left it all behind to marry a prince, and the world applauded her for delivering us a real-life fairy tale. The trade-off was obvious and in keeping with worldly values.

Machel Shull is different; she found the excess and superficiality of that life made her feel hollow inside. In that realization she discovered that no material thing or outer success could ever make her happy, so she chose to look for the treasures within.

In *Live Love Soul* Machel has written a very liberating book which acts as a roadmap for tapping into the wellspring of peace, joy and happiness that is freely available to us all, no matter what your outer circumstance may be. This book is about living in the now and waking up to appreciate how wonderful and magnificent you are. It inspires you to fulfill your dreams while remaining steadfast and connected to a world that needs your kindness, compassion and humility.

The author is indeed a very happy woman who loves and lives life to the fullest; from the solitary delight of a morning sunrise, to a holiday replete with extended family and a menagerie of creatures, from Doberman Pinschers to peacocks. Most of all, Machel is a big-hearted, luminous soul who loves to inspire other women to discover their greatest potential, even when that means looking at your darker shadow side, owning and loving it, since this is the way we fully self-actualize as complete human beings.

In her previous book, *Middle Age Beauty*, the author inspires us to grow older and wiser with each birthday; to enter into a deep, loving relationship with respect for ourselves and without

1

recourse to Botox or plastic surgery. This book urges the reader to go deeper; to live from the place of your heart and discover the passion that lights a fire in your belly. In this way you are invited to become the hero of your own story, like a warrior princess, who is capable of building her own kingdom from the inside out.

Machel in no way romanticizes this journey. In fact, she clearly states that determination and stamina are needed if you wish to acquire the ultimate prize of attaining your dreams. Often a shift in perception is needed to stir oneself from comfortable self-defeatist thoughts and attitudes to a new belief that *yes, no matter how many times I fail, I will get up and start again*.

All throughout *Live Love Soul* Machel does not hold back on sharing with us insights from the high and low points of her own story. She tells us of her struggles and of how she learned to prepare her soul for both victory and defeat. She says, "If something hurts deeply, reach for the tiny joys you have discovered that can make your heart sing, to lean on during the tough times."

The author imparts her wisdom in a chatty, friendly manner reminiscent of a big sister inspiring a younger sibling to love and believe in herself. Though written in a light-hearted manner, this book has the power to totally transform your life. Enjoy.

~ **Mary Elizabeth Coen,** International Bestselling Author of *Love and the Goddess*

Your energy can defeat you, but your soul will make you win.
~ William Ray Penn

Dwell on the beauty of life. Watch the stars, and see yourself running with them.
~ Marcus Aurelius

Dear Readers

During my mid-twenties I hit upon a major stumbling block on my journey. When I turned 25, I remember looking around in my Los Angeles setting wondering about the 'big picture' in life. Instead of looking for a good time with my friends and booking acting and modeling auditions, I found that there was something fundamentally missing from my inner world. After a confident beginning at the age of 18, I thought I had the world at my feet and knew everything. I thought this was going to be such a simple journey. Oh, how I was wrong.

But that morning when I turned 25, I felt an overwhelming feeling of sadness and angst. I lived in an A-frame guesthouse in the middle of Studio City just about 5 miles away from Universal Studios. I remember that morning like it was yesterday. I woke up feeling like I had isolated myself in this tiny cabin and I wasn't quite sure how my road had led me there.

My steps and the confidence of my youth had led me to a place that I had never been before: a blank page and an uncertain future that I did not understand.

After chasing dreams and following my creativity and achieving decent success, the bottom fell out. The world felt flat and my soul felt empty. I tried to talk to my friends about this new feeling. You know, a new awakening from within that wanted more than just instant gratification from a fun night out on Sunset Boulevard or booking another commercial with the cameras rolling. I needed something with deeper meaning. What was missing? Why wasn't I happy?

From that day forward, I can look back and see my journey of wanting to discover: What makes me happy and why? How can I be happy right now?

What is happiness?

And how can I be happy when I don't always get what I want?

This quest led me to my best journey so far...*my journey within*. This book is essentially my story of ups and downs. My ins and outs and how what I have found out is happiness can also be a matter of living better, loving more correctly, and sharing and uncovering my own soul. My journey led me to discover 'little things' I can do each day to change my world and make my own happiness. I discovered I loved running. So I became a runner. I discovered that I loved books. So I started reading more. I discovered that I loved rollerblading. So I went out to this golf course in the Valley with a 10-mile path of sidewalk strip, so I could blissfully feel the wind beating down on my face as I whisked side to side in my rollerblades. I got busy finding out what makes me happy.

I remember one of my managers at my part-time position at the Sunset Marquis Hotel saying, "You must be in love, you look so happy, Machel. New boyfriend?"

"No...I am just happy."

"Really? Wow. Whatever you are doing, it shows!"

I walked away with the best smile that day. How great that all my efforts were actually showing on the outside, too! So I kept my nose to the grindstone. I kept unearthing new ways to discover how to achieve a sense of well-being without being specifically attached to an outcome.

I worked on meditation. I studied self-help books. I hung out with actors late at night and discussed our fondest desires. I took time to enjoy my coffee in the morning. I watched the birds take flight and land on the branches in front of the little cabin I lived in, nestled in the suburban neighborhood. I found a life coach. I studied Norman Vincent Peale's many 'power of positive thinking' books that empowered my mind, changed my thoughts and lifted my temporary cloud of depression. That yellow brick falling from the sky that had side-swiped me on my 25th birthday had been decimated by active efforts of fighting for that smile I thought was rightfully mine.

I took time to get to know myself over the years. Even as my life changed and I moved to a different city, I took what I learned with me. I stayed connected to the joys of right now. Life is always a challenge of trying to balance our schedules, do what we must, while finding some much-needed fun along the way, too.

Some may think that a bubbly personality lacks a bit of reality. I say, wake up and grab that smile! Plow your way through to the joy you deserve. Fight those defeatists; don't listen to the naysayers.

Dig in and make this your rosy mad-capped day. Bee-bop your head. Drink tea. Watch the birds. Force a laugh...*fight* for your happiness. Don't be a sourpuss. You deserve to feel good from the inside out and discover what makes your soul gleam with love.

This book is about living more, loving more and sharing more of your soul. It's about uncovering how you can find happiness at your fingertips every day even if you are fighting depression.

It's not a destination. It's not a goal. It's not what we can have when we achieve something fantastic. It's a mood that feels strong, calm and grounded from within the inner recesses of your soul that bubbles to the surface at a pleasant cadence. This book is about finding happiness NOW in your current situation and being grateful for your blessings.

Life can be short. We cannot always change what surrounds us. We cannot undo what is behind us. We cannot predict the future. But we can wake up and take charge of our surroundings and be the captain of our own life and be the Rock Star of our own show.

So I am asking you, dear reader, are you ready to uncover simple ways to define what brings you happiness? If so, let's take this journey together through these pages.

Oh, and on the most important note! I am so thrilled to have interviewed some fantastic individuals who share with me their personal secrets on ways to stay passionate and in love with life. One is a famous violinist. Another is a snowboarder; we also meet an author and Zen meditation coach, two doctors, a matchmaker and an international bestselling author from Ireland. All of their stories are so fascinating. From snowboarding down the highest mountain peaks to performing to sold-out crowds across the world, I am sure you will love hearing what these true rock star individuals have to say. They share their passion, dreams and secrets inside these pages with you and me.

So let's get busy and discover ways to bring you more joy each day on your own journey.

Sincerely,

~ Machel

PS: My name is pronounced like Michelle. And just so I don't have to endure the misspelling of my name at every coffee shop, I simply go by my nickname *Mimi*.

Introduction

Who am I? I am a person just like you who lives every day looking for moments of bliss and happiness. While some might believe that inner happiness is linked to your wallet or your car size, *Live Love Soul* can help you identify moments during your routine that can enhance your daily activities and improve your mood. How? By submitting simple suggestions that can trigger moments of bliss, little joys and inner joy without looking for another person or an outside circumstance to do this for you.

As I described, dear reader, in the beginning I had to go within, do my homework and grasp onto the fundamentals of simple things to alleviate and pull my soul back into the sunlight. How do we survive and find a way to go on if what we love is suddenly gone? How do we take moments to rebuild joy if there seems to be a never-ending burden wearing on our soul? We have to take baby steps back into the light, and make a *concerted effort* to find the light again.

Where Is the Soul?

This is a question worth investigating and applying to our own lives. Is it in eating organic? Is it watching the *Today Show* early in the morning? Is it hanging out with your friends? This book will help you break down simple facts, triggers and routines that can keep you more connected to the most important person you need to be taking care of right now…*you*. The trick is to know who you are and what nourishes your inner soul first. Can you say that you know what that is for yourself? If you can only answer a timid 'yes', now is the time to map out and create your best world by discovering more about yourself and developing an inner life with your soul.

So how do we do that? How do you connect to the soul when your everyday life is tempting you moment by moment to stay entertained, less inspired, and wired into what the latest upgrade in technology will be? You don't want to miss the moment of *now* because you are too busy adding that fabulous photo of the sunset you took just as it melted across the horizon to your favorite social networking site. Trust me, I am guilty of this, too. I must step away from electronic gadgets and become more present. This is a question that I pondered while writing another book, *Middle Age Beauty*. In it, I break down an important equation that outlines Soul, Health, and Beauty. The number one factor that adds to true beauty comes from within us all.

When we can identify our purpose and meaning from the inside, we can find a much more exciting and rewarding experience *now*. We must discover what treasures are ours for the taking. Are you taking time to do that now with yourself? Do you know what connects your inner heart to that one desire that makes you feel passionate and alive?

I will take you through some fabulous interviews with individuals who have devoted time and study to developing ways to unearth their own happiness and what their soulful life resembles. Find out ways to discover how to get connected to your inner dreams. But most importantly: *Are you having fun being with just yourself?*

Live

Every moment and every event of every man's life on earth plants something in his soul.
~ Thomas Merton

Part One—Live will examine easy methods and exercises that will help you feel more grounded, peaceful, while living in the midst of your current lifestyle. Are you working at a job you don't necessarily love? Are you feeling exhausted? Are you unsure of why there is any hope worth living for out on the horizon? Have you experienced a recent shift that has caused you turmoil, hurt or uncertainty? How do you find a direction if you feel hopeless? Living every day is something we do no matter what. Are you attacking the week with a plan or does each week just sort of string on to the next? In this section, we will tackle simple exercises that can help you redirect your steps.

Interviews: Jeremy Jones and Dr Jason Karp. These two inspiring individuals will definitely motivate you to find more time out in nature that involves exercise and soul-nourishing moments…not to mention *adventure*!

Love

Love makes your soul crawl out from its hiding place.
~ Zora Neale Hurston

Part Two—Love will take on that all-encompassing, powerful emotion that we are all seeking always, *love*. In this section, I will share with you some of my own vulnerable times and reveal to you the soulful secrets that I apply each day to increase my own level of compassion, caring and gratitude. While we know it's great to love and to find compassion, how can we do it, if we feel angered or are constantly wanting to judge others? If our innate nature is prone to measure up others with a sharp and unkind eye, what can we do to break down this thought process? Discover an applicable tip that can help break the cycle of summing up and judging others. Find out ways to enhance your weekly schedule with activities that will re-energize your soul. And, when all else fails, you must do *this* to find love…what could that be?

Interviews: Elle France, co-founder of SingldOut matchmaking site, shares relationship basics in the romance department. Mary

Elizabeth Coen, the international bestselling author of *Love and the Goddess*, shares her personal inspiring story of how she pursued her dreams of becoming a bestselling author and redefining her own self-love.

Soul

Certain springs are tapped only when we are alone.
~ Anne Morrow Lindbergh

Part Three—Soul is the section that will help you discover and make time for inner moments of solitude. Why should we do this? You can help heal, learn and improve the quality of your daily life. Maybe it's 5 minutes, maybe it's 20...you will see there are many ways you can squeeze in a 'peaceful Zen zone' that will ultimately improve your mental and personal health. Your soul is counting on you to learn how to be more attentive and reflective. This section is dedicated to helping you understand the value of a 'quiet, reflective space' and how to tap into the inner recesses of your soul.

Interviews: World-renowned violinist Lindsey Stirling shares in an intimate interview how she found inner courage to pursue her dream as a solo rock violinist. Her performances have sold out worldwide and she shares what inspires her to keep on believing in her dreams.

Dr Doris McCoy has traveled the world searching for 'the happiest place on earth.' You might be surprised by her findings. She shares with you her passion for positivity and believing in our 'natural right' to be happy.

How to Use This Book
Feel free to mark up the pages in this book for your exercises. Mark the corners with dog-ears, read the last chapter first, skip

around, or read it from start to finish. It's up to you. But ultimately, besides sharing my own stories and struggles that have helped me find more inspiration and happiness, I discovered that life is much like school. Sometimes we need to do our homework to experience the joy of living our best. So here are some simple things I will ask you to grab at the end of some of the chapters.

What you will need:

- A yoga mat or a large resting pillow; a beach towel could work, too
- An empty box with a cover (you can buy a cute craft box for under $10.00!)
- Pen and paper
- A blank journal
- A quiet space where you can easily make time to do this weekly

The beginning of discovering your own beautiful soul starts with you.

One of my favorite authorities on positivity and living a better quality of life was Dr Norman Vincent Peale. He once said, "If you want things to be different, perhaps the answer is to become different yourself." His advice may seem impossible and we may just think, "That's just the way I am naturally."

Not so.

Live Love Soul will guide you with daily activities so you can step into your own dynamic world where you deserve to be living. It doesn't matter how old you are. You can create a new 'you' at any age.

In the inspiring and all-knowing words of the famous aviator, celebrity, mother and author Anne Morrow Lindbergh, who said it best:

The final answer, I know, is always inside. But the outside can give a clue, can help one to find the answer. One is free, like the hermit crab, to change one's shell.

So soak up those words of wisdom. Don't look back in 20 years with regrets. Make time now to live a more exciting and fulfilling life. Your soul is waiting for you...

Part One — Live

Life moves pretty fast. If you don't stop and look around once in a while, you could miss it.
~ John Hughes, *Ferris Bueller's Day Off*

Many people lose the small joys in the hope for the big happiness.
~ Pearl S. Buck, Nobel Prize winner

Chapter 1

Oh, the Small Joys

Lately, I have been big on these *small joys* in life. Yes, you know the kind. A good cup of tea, cozy flannel pajamas and a thick wordy book for a Saturday evening alone. A tiny trick to find happiness is to cultivate the 'small joys,' and make time for little blissful moments throughout your week. What will this require? What makes you happy? What little rituals, tiny things or moments can you go to, to improve your overall sense of well-being?

Here is my quick list that's bound to get my joy level rocking:

- An early morning run
- Walking my dog around the block
- Music in my car lined up—Lady Gaga, One Republic, Lindsey Stirling, Thirty Seconds to Mars
- A trip to the bookstore
- Bird-watching in the morning
- A nature hike
- Chatting with my girlfriends on the phone
- Calling my sister or mom for a long phone conversation
- Making a vegetable and fruit juice in my juicer
- A coffee shop stop (my favorite just happens to be Peets Coffee)
- Spending cozy time with my fur babies
- Acting incredibly goofy in my car, while I am jamming out to music

I keep my little life busy with personal tasks of moments that I know can infuse my soul with some joy. I schedule them. I make them happen. I wake up with an attitude of, "This is it! Let's make today count." Well, I'm not always zany happy, but I set the wheels in motion so those 'organic moments of bliss' can funnel out on some level that day.

For example, in the mornings I have my cup of coffee in my *favorite* coffee mug, while watching the birds eat the birdseed in my tiny backyard. I relax. I enjoy the actual taste of the coffee. I savor the smell, the temperature and the way it feels when I hold my coffee cup in my hands. I am capturing a small joy for the beginning of my day. I am sitting there in my pajamas in the early morning light, not being disturbed by anyone or anything. On the days I start off like this, I can observe usually my mood is more upbeat. I feel more relaxed and not rushed because I made time for 'me.' (This will be a theme throughout the book. Making time for you.)

I also take time to read books. I take time to take breaks from my goals, my deadlines, my friendships and time that might prevent me from feeling soulful. I make time for that soulful stuff. I make it my mission. I place it first. I don't want to just be pushing and pulling for the next achievement, minute, moment. No. I want to be relaxing down to the core of my bones by unraveling what makes my soul feel most comfortable.

Why is this important to do? You must prepare your soul for victories and defeats

If you learn to cultivate your own soulful life, these steps can protect you and help you recover from the harder moments or the disappointments. If something hurts deeply, reach for the tiny joys you have discovered that can make your heart sing, to lean on during the tough times. What makes you tick? What do you love? Don't stay lost or distracted in another person. Don't stay glued to the gossip. Relax and step away. Discover some non-attachment time. You might be surprised by what you find if you go digging around in the deep recesses of your untapped soul. You could discover a new hobby, an invention, a new career, a business, something that just sets your life on fire that had been missing.

So make some ME time. It's good to relax and breathe

Don't be too sad if you miss that one party you thought you could go to. Don't worry. Another special occasion will come your way. You can make something new happen for yourself every day. One of my favorite quotes ever is by Norman Vincent Peale. This quote has pulled me through the darkest hours, outlining a ray of hope just sparkling on the shoreline, just in reach of my next dream: "Don't let your circumstances defeat you. Be bigger than your circumstances." Something like that anyway.

I liked how he laid it out. As if yes, indeed, life can be a game. You win or you lose. And in the end it is up to us. *What defines us, what breaks us, what molds us, what person do we want to shine for the world to see? What mark are you hoping to make in this life for yourself or your family?*

These are important things to ponder. So set your party hat down. Don't go out with your friends every night. Take some quiet time away from your children or your partner and make a few moments for yourself.

Just make sure to go light on your feet

Think happy thoughts. Stave off those dreaded negative words that make you feel like nothing. The world is in need of a 'better YOU.' Figure out what your 'go-to' joyful moments can be, so you can schedule them, lean on them and have little things to look forward to. You may never win that trip to Fiji. You may never win an Oscar.

And so what? That is not the life you were meant to live. You are here now. So make the most of your surroundings. Don't play the 'compare game.' Just work on yourself and what you can do *now*. So in the meantime, cultivate, study and find out what makes you...what? *Happy!*

Even a happy life cannot be without a measure of darkness, and the word 'happy' would lose its meaning if it were not balanced by sadness. It is far better to take things as they come along with patience and equanimity.

~ Carl Jung

Chapter 2

This Too Shall Pass

Sometimes life takes us down. We become ill. The weather is subzero with a negative wind-chill of minus 45. The driver in front of you is driving 10 miles under the speed limit and you may run late for that important meeting. Your neighbors are remodeling their home...*again*. Meanwhile you are shopping at second-hand shops and are thrilled with your next bath rug. You look for love on the Internet via Facebook friends. They are all posting about politics, memes and cats, and more cats. We look for inspiration and there is none to find. You may find yourself wishing you were that celebrity who just came back from Tahiti. Their sunbaked tan and flip flops with million-dollar shades in their 'selfies' on Instagram leave you feeling bitter. You may feel like, "Why them and not me?"

"When is it my turn?" you might be thinking.

Why can life be so uneven and not what I was expecting? I put out the effort and my results have been slim.

The Truth

This world owes you nothing. This life is not a bargain, a ride, a gift or a shopping spree. It's your day-to-day grind of you figuring out how to make the moments count. You could be juggling two careers, a side job and raising three kids. You might be unemployed and your bumper was just smashed in by an uninsured motorist. There might be a chance your relatives are living it up, while you seem to be constantly in a struggle or even worse—on a downward spiral. What can we do when the world feels like something worse than a cheap knock-off of an Andy Warhol pop-art painting?

Hang in there. This moment won't last. It's temporary. These

21

feelings will subside and there is a chance that if you are on a downward spiral, your time to change is just around the corner.

Sometimes the world is gray. The sky is black. Terrible things happen. Unjustly, wrongs happen daily and we wonder why that reality star is raking in the bucks as they sip giant margaritas. Sometimes life doesn't make sense. These outer circumstances that do not define or touch your life should not in any way bring you to a deep sadness. No. Rather reflect on the incongruent nature and let it go. You will have enough to worry about in your own life without letting things on the Internet bring you down.

However, at this moment as I write this, I am in my worst-looking teal flannel pajamas with a stain on the right corner. My hair is in a messy bun. I have been 'coughing up a lung' for the last week and languishing in a sickness that has knocked me sideways. When we get sick, the world feels dim. Life turns down a few notches and nothing that we cared about seems to matter.

When this happens, what can you do?

We must remind ourselves, 'This Too Shall Pass.' So if you are experiencing a real lull on your journey, pause and remember it won't be forever.

I remember only a few years ago, two of my close friends died within 6 months of each other. The world had never seemed grimmer, less extraordinary or less magical. My grief was deep and wide. I had never felt such pain that could tip over my normal day in life. Each day felt heavy, clouded, and it was almost a burden to breathe. I switched my jobs. Worked as a receptionist for a garage door company and happily answered phones in the quiet space of the showroom. I had to shift my world in order to deal with the grief properly. I needed to shut down and to reflect on my emotions. This new environment, though not sexy or career zappy, was just what my soul needed.

But with much downtime and solace and reflection, I allowed myself to grieve. I did not run from my emotions, but instead embraced them wholeheartedly. This life is but a vapor and we can either choose to experience it all or numb ourselves to the pain.

What is important to know is there will be a reprieve. Yes! A break or a shift in your reality. Life can take a sudden mystical turn you had no way of foreseeing. Sometimes the best-laid secrets are the ones we cannot see. They lie just around the corner in the mystery of life.

These moments of aches and pains, sickness, disease, distress and grief can shift for us. When we least expect it, there will be a break in the clouds. We will be able to see a new direction we could not see before.

So if you are guessing, yes, as I write this, I have had one of those days. One of those days when I felt like nothing and life felt rather grim. I noticed the sun kept on shining though. I kept on walking. I kept on thinking, "This…too…shall…pass." We can't always be sunshine and rainbows. There has to be a down period so we can recognize the joy when it hits us full throttle.

So take this time to do a little exercise with me. I would like you to write yourself a letter. And in this letter, I would like you to tell your inner 'self': *It's okay, I will allow myself to have a break from being on top, from feeling joy, from being inspiring, or from sharing the joy. Today is just not that day.*

Exercise: Write a letter to yourself. Set up your quiet space. Roll out your yoga pad or grab a soft blanket so you can sit and write freely in your quiet space. This space is important to create so you can become more centered and rooted to your deeper thoughts.

Here is an example of my letter:

Dear Me,
The world is not perfect and neither are you. This day feels like nothing and today that is okay. It's okay to be human. To

feel sad, to feel low and to feel like this life just really adds up to some anguish and pain. This life feels like it hurts too much and I am mad about that. I am mad about all the hurts and pains that I cannot take away from this life, change or heal. I am mad at my own inadequacies. But today is a PJ Day, a sick day. A day of rest. A day of reconciliation. A day to be angry. A day to be mad. A day to let bygones be left in the past. I can't do it all every day perfectly. Sometimes this life is too much. So take a breather on me and relax. Don't take it all so seriously. Breathe. Do some breathing exercises. Imagine your favorite place and visit it in your mind. Be free of your surroundings that confine you. Don't be so hard on yourself.

There is time for rest. This day is for you. There is time for being a disheveled mess. This day is for you. Tomorrow might be that day when your sunshine comes back. You know, the spark in your step that tells you, "You are a Rock Star!"

But today, give it a rest. Read a book. Take a break from the Internet. Don't call your friends. Don't call your family. Just take some time to heal. This day is just for you. You have earned it.

Thank you for listening and for relaxing and for shutting out the monkey chatter of mean words. Because really, I deserve love. I deserve you to love me even when I am at my weakest…

Signed ~ Machel

Your Task

Write out a letter to yourself with kind and loving words. Buy a little wooden box or creative paper box to place next to your bed. Leave the letter there for trying times and read it when you need it. Buy little gold stars and keep them in the box, too. When you need to read the letter and you apply and help change your attitude for the better, give yourself a *gold star*! You deserve it. This may seem childish. But our soul still loves to be rewarded with little things that make us smile from the inside out.

Remember the world can be brutal. Stay good to yourself and speak kinds words to your soul.

Because after all, there is no such thing as a perfect life. The green grass on the other side of the fence may just be Astroturf. Don't be fooled by the glitter. Make your own backyard beautiful. And if you are having a bad day, give yourself a break and be kind to your soul.

Life belongs to the living, and he who lives must be prepared for changes.
~ Johann Wolfgang von Goethe

Chapter 3

Don't Leave Home without These Three Things

Right now I am sitting in a Starbucks in a suburb of San Diego watching a young mother look gleefully fulfilled, while her 4-year-old son with the perfect haircut and summer striped shirt is longingly adoring her from across the tiny round table. There is another baby next to her with his legs propped up on the outside of the baby jogger. His face and body are neatly tucked inside for his perfect nap as his young momma clocks a few moments of dreaminess inside an air-conditioned Starbucks in the semi-desert area of Southern California.

This mom at the moment has found temporary bliss. A purpose. A meaning. A reason to get out of bed and make her world flow with love and compassion for the children she is raising. Of course if this is it for her, at some point she will maybe need a hobby or two to fulfill that mid-life 'empty nester' syndrome. She is wearing yoga shorts and a workout top with Nikes. She looks rather fit, so I am sure this is one of her bonus perks, too, that add that gleam to her eye. I am happy to sit here and watch this sweet moment. It reminds me of me with my son when he was little. Now he is a teenager. I couldn't be more proud of him. But those adoring eyes have turned to, "Mom, can you just give me a little peace, please? You need to learn how to be at peace with yourself. You don't need to talk all the time to me. It's okay to be silent." Big words for a 14-year-old. Maybe he's got a point.

My son has hit a nerve with me that brings me to this chapter. And that little private moment I was witnessing at Starbucks is now over. The mother has gone and now the chairs are empty. A little nostalgia courses through my thoughts as I type this. A sense of sadness at the passage of time that keeps passing. We make moments that will turn into memories. Days will pass. This day may be forgotten for that mother at this Starbucks. There are so many that weave a tapestry for her family…

This is the story of our life. This is the way life goes. We spend our minutes and hours as they unfold into an ending of a new day. How we spend each waking moment is at the tip of our fingers and inside the well of our souls.

So how are you going to spend your time on this earth? As my son is growing up and needing me less, I find myself aching for that sweet little boy who adored me. I know he still does…the point is my happiness needs to first be rooted within myself and my soul in order to grow.

The question is: are you spending your time in a way that *will add* happiness to your life? Are you living the dream you had as a child? Or are you just marking time because you have let go of your wishes because you have been convinced by the jaded aspect of society that this is just the way life goes? Don't let this life strip you of your enthusiasm! Fight for it and demand to find that 'special something' that gives your inner world more purpose and meaning.

So how do we do this? Let's make a check list, shall we? Let's get down to business.

In order to spend our time wisely and happily, there are a few important items to check off the list:

- Do you love where you live?
- Are you happy with the relationships in your life?
- Do you like your current job or the career you are in?
- Do you have a hobby that brings you daily bliss or something you can look forward to a few times a week?
- Are you keeping your life on a schedule or is it sort of a fly-by-the-seat-of-your-pants type of affair, snowballing into

the unexpected?

So now write down your list. Write down your answers. Do you like what you see? If you don't, do not fret! This life is yours for the taking! Tomorrow, as Scarlett O'Hara so appropriately said at the end of *Gone With the Wind*,

After all, tomorrow is another day.

Now what you need is your arsenal of supplies to help you tackle, guide and live the life you want to live. Are you ready? Are you ready to map out the life you are supposed to be living? Your soul deserves to be happy. If you aren't, there is a good chance you may need to redirect your thoughts and harness them inward to detect where you are off in your footing.

This might require a life coach. This might require a counselor. Or maybe you have a good connection to quiet and prayer time that can help guide you through the darkest of waters. So first ask yourself this if you aren't living the life you wish you were: how do I get back on track?

Should I reach out for help?

My little back story—which if you read *Middle Age Beauty* you will know—is that I gained much help and guidance in my late twenties when I needed to redirect my path and discover new dreams. I went to church every Sunday at 5 p.m. at this gorgeous cathedral church in Studio City. I found a therapist that I trusted. And I enlisted a Zen life coach. Yes, call me desperate if you will. Make fun of me. Shout to the mountain tops, "Goodness, that girl needed help!" And you are right to throw your stones.

I did.

I had the courage to seek it, to find a better answer, and that is what we must do when we need to start over. Have the courage to seek help. Not from your friends. Not from a family member, but from an outside source that can help bolster your confidence, help you find your way back to the happy life you deserve to be living.

So don't be afraid. Therapy helps us sift through the dirt of our past and helps us understand the mistakes we continue to keep making. Yes, "the forest for the trees" quote applies here.

If you can't afford therapy, you can always seek counseling through a local spiritual organization. You could also check out Learning Annex classes for a new perspective. My best advice would be to humble yourself. Ask for help. Find those knees and a prayer for guidance in your heart.

A silent prayer can open a new porthole to untapped discoveries.

Now that you have done that, sought guidance if you need it, make sure you are armed with the right supplies that can help you tackle this life. Many times we start our day without proper food or rest from the night before. So how can we ever expect to have a shiny day if we aren't taking proper care of ourselves?

Think of the marathoner about to start a 26.2 mile journey. Do you think they arrived at the moment on the start line without great preparation or the tools to help them combat their training period before their marathon? Do you know that many of them pack food, sports gels, gummy bears, candies, protein bars...those little things their body needs to help power them over the finish line? These runners don't go at it alone. They are prepared, trained and ready. Life requires us to take ample action for our dreams to materialize. Otherwise our dreams are just sawdust on the floor. The same is true on our journey. We need the right arsenal of supplies so we can take action and make our goals have 'lift-off wings.'

These supplies aren't something you can touch with your fingertips. These three supplies are *key components* for whether or not you can figure out how to be happier. You will need them. You will need to arm your thoughts, your prayers and your daily rituals with these three spiritual warrior tools. They are ones that you have heard of before. But there is a reason. *You need them* to make it through the hills and valleys. The sad times, the good times, those unexpected shocking circumstances you never saw coming.

You need these three in your battle for carving out your right to be happy:

Faith

What is faith? Faith is the ability to believe in something you cannot see. It's a feeling that grounds you with spiritual roots. Faith will build your confidence. You must apply faith to unseen dreams and places and things you do not see but can feel in your heart. You steadily keep this seed of faith (yes, like that mustard seed!) planted deep within your soul to help you navigate through uncharted waters. You use faith to build one more baby step as a solution to your problems. You use faith to restore the bitterness that can impede our hearts.

The late, great Dr Norman Vincent Peale's books revolutionized and changed my thinking patterns. The greatest gift of all his messages had to be on faith. He had one simple exercise that he gave his readers:

Act as if and it shall be.
~ Norman Vincent Peale

I applied this simple principle to little areas in my life and saw immediate results. An example would be when you wake up in the morning. If you tend to be a grouch, act as if you feel happy. Do this repeatedly for many days in a row. Eventually it will sink in and you will feel what you are suggesting to your mind 'to be.' Our thoughts are powerful. We can shape our daily moments with laser-beam thinking. And with the power of faith behind it, anything is possible.

Courage

Courage is the ability to have strength during challenging or frightening times. This quality we can develop in our lives. Courage is asking yourself to 'be brave' when fear is the obvious first thing we feel. Courage is what we need to build bridges over hard times, bereavement, and times of depression when our mind feels like it's stuck in a dark hole. The very act of courage can help you achieve your dreams and the happiness you are seeking. When we do what we need to do, this can be, in fact, a simple courageous act of 'doing what must be done.' One of my favorite mantras ever that I still live by is a quote by Goethe:

Do what must be done. This may not be happiness, but it is greatness.

What I have discovered is that by applying this quote and completing actions, the effect ends up being happiness because you are doing what you need to do in order to have and live a better life.

Every day may not be a vacation to a tropical island or blissful moments at a spa with two cucumbers covering our eyes, while our feet are being massaged by candlelight. Bliss and happiness can come from doing those nitty-gritty things that need to get done, like cleaning, studying for that test, doing your work after working hours, or adding an extra hour of time with your children because they need their momma. All of these things may sound small. Ordinary. And maybe boring. Just remember, it takes great courage to live an exemplary ordinary life. To live one in peace of mind, happiness and in spirit.

Your destiny may not be jet-setting across the continents to be on a safari in Africa. Your destiny might be right where you are—*now*. Doing what must be done and living a good, simple and fulfilling ordinary life. So have courage in your ordinary daily life. Have courage through the hard times. Do those little things that must be done and seeds of happiness will blossom in your heart.

Hope

Have hope in your dreams. Hope is not a noun. It's a verb. It's an action. A feeling that you can transcend to the core of your soul and help you power out your future or what you are wanting to happen in your life. Developing the ability to 'have hope' in your dreams can dispel fear or insecurities. This may be your most important one to have in the arsenal of your spiritual supplies. Apply this verb to your heart and make your mark on this world. What do you hope for? Maybe it is as simple as 'having courage and having faith' to be the person you want to be. Maya Angelou's thoughts on hope exemplify the ordinary moments in life that need hope to attain what our hearts desire:

> My great hope is to laugh as much as I cry; to get my work done and try to love somebody and have the courage to accept the love in return.

I like this quote. I love her wisdom. I hope I can embrace her words and apply them to my here and now.

That earlier Starbucks moment with the mother enjoying being 'a mom' to her son has faded. The day has folded over into the afternoon. I am sitting here at my husband's family's produce business listening to the humming of the cars pass by. I can smell the fresh strawberries for sale in front of me. I can feel the gentle breeze against my face. Robin is speaking to someone about their passion, which I am not kidding just happens to be meditating. He is telling us about this website on how to download talks on 'how to meditate better.' I smile inwardly to myself at how perfect this day has been. So simple with moments that mean so much to the mother and her son, to me, the observer, and now a customer just looking for a simple piece of happiness. These are the small things worth noticing. Life has the most beautiful moments laid out before us. We just need to tune in and be more observant.

To find these moments and to honor them, we need to carve out our own moments of bliss. And in order to do that, we need to keep those three important components close to our heart: *faith, courage* and *hope*. This life trickles forward into the next moment and the next. The trick is to have the courage to be present now, so we can experience the beauty that surrounds us.

Comparison is the thief of joy.
~ Theodore Roosevelt

Chapter 4

Bloom Where You Are Planted on Independence Day

Today is the 4th of July. I am sitting on a hard metal chair next to my Doberman. He is now going on 2 years old. We are with my husband today at his family's business, which is a local farm and produce shop in Southern California. I think most associate the Fourth of July with fireworks, watermelon and parades. But today my holiday is here at my husband's business in Southern California, helping the customers find their last-minute items for their barbecue. Corn is a favorite. Our chocolate-dipped covered strawberries are world famous. At least in the area where we live. And right now a young lady with a cool-looking Hollywood hat is giving the heirloom tomatoes a thorough check, before she decides on which one to buy for her salad later this evening.

In the past, in my younger years, there might have been a smaller voice in me crying out, "But it's the Fourth of July, baby. Do we have to open?" However, after seven years of being married to a farmer (well, not technically, but definitely a gardener), I have come to realize that holidays at the produce shop are the best days to be open. So a holiday to the rest of the world may equal a busy workday at the fruit-stand.

While my friends are drinking in the bright golden sun just a few miles down at the beach, I count myself lucky to be here. I count myself lucky to count the small blessings that are actually larger than real life in some ways.

In this chapter I am going to share with you four important factors for how to avoid the 'comparison is thief' trap, which we can so easily fall prey to, and steer you close to happier moments in your world. They may seem like the obvious, yet it's an everyday life of being busy where these four simple things we do—traits—can rob us of our moments of bliss just at the base of our fingertips.

Comparing Your Life to Others

With the recent surge in glamorous reality shows with skinny housewives that look almost too perfect and somewhat plastic, and the shows where you've got those bearded folks selling all kinds of home goods in Walmart to a pawnshop broker raking in the dough, your life may feel a little boring. Hey, this is me, too. After living in Hollywood and running that circuit for a bit, you could say my initial reaction to San Diego was a rather big river of tears of, "What am I going to do here?" And that dreaded of all fears: is my life going to be boring? Ahh. The fear, the agony in that. Maybe this is not a fear of yours. But it has always been mine. Maybe that's why I keep myself active and busy. I like being interested in where I am, to love what I am doing and find excitement under the ordinary.

So today is a day when my heart wants to think obvious thoughts: "Wish we were at those beach parties we were invited to..." But the reality is I am here with my husband, my most cherished loved one walking the planet, besides my son and immediate family members. So how can you beat that?

I looked most of my life for this man (well, not always looking, but hoping) and here he is and my life is with him...and if that means I'm in the fruit and vegetable business on Independence Day, I think I can swing this.

The reality is I go all week knowing my holiday won't be capped off with bubbles and beers at the beach. More like hanging out with organic fruits and cheerful customers. So I start planting my seeds of success for a good day. I imagine it happy, peaceful and quiet. I got up extra early, too, to get my run in the neighborhood and then drove my son to one of the beach parties. At least he was able to go. Now I am here. I am thinking about the significance of *why* 'comparison is thief' and why it's important to stop doing that to ourselves.

Here is a list to think about and apply to your life:

1. Where you are, if it's not what you love, you have the ability to change it in the future. So still be thankful for where you are and for your blessings. Build a better tomorrow and count your blessings today. So don't be wishing the day away for better things to come. Today is the first day of the rest of your life. So have FUN wherever you are on your journey. Hang tight and don't be a baby.

2. Make time for special moments to make your day better. Do you love coffee or tea? So buy that special mug to brighten your day. Carry it with you like a security blanket to remind you of one happy thing you have in your hand. (Yes, this works! But be careful. I have dropped a couple of my cherished ones in the past. The good news is they are relatively inexpensive.)

3. Smile and be happy anyway. By placing your positivity into your thoughts, you can actually shift your feeling with aggressive positive thinking. That's right. Get busy and think that this world and where you are is excellent! YOU are excellent. Give yourself a pat on the back and remind yourself this is just one day in your life. Forget that it may be your birthday and you are all alone. Forget that this could be the holiday season and you are going through a bad break-up. Instead, turn your alone time into your own 'upbeat party' with a positive force that will be reckoned with... When you step into an office or building, the immediate effect might be one of, "Wow, she is so chipper! I wish I could be that happy." Yep! You can zing strangers with that happy, zippy step that leaves them in a warm glow.

4. *Be present* with the present. Don't avoid where you are. Make the most of it. Enjoy the challenge of making your day great. You can do it! Don't be a baby. Buck *up*, as they say in the

Midwest in the US, and don't let yourself down by being ungrateful for your immediate surroundings. Someone down the street or your next-door neighbor could be dealing with far worse circumstances. Dr Norman Vincent Peale once said in one of his books, "Be thankful for the ability to write with a pencil and to move your hands." Lovely. Simple and so true. 'Be thankful' are the two key words there.

Back to 'Bloom where you are planted…' I do believe that is a Mary Engelbreit quote. I have always loved her art and inspirational messages. Do that. Yes, *bloom* where you are in this life. You may be dreaming of Greece, Spain or some exotic island, but you live among rows of corn in the Midwest or maybe you are surrounded by mountains. Utilize and enjoy where you are.

Don't keep thinking thoughts like these:

- If I could just move here, I would be happy.
- If I could just change jobs or get that job promotion, then I would be happy.
- If I could just marry this one guy I am in love with, I would be happy.
- If I could just get this one girl to love me, I would be happy.
- If I could start a Facebook business and go public like Mark Zuckerberg, I would be happy.

You get the drift. STOP thinking thoughts like this. Instead you need to internalize and identify exactly what your blessings are and start counting them on a daily basis.

Practice gratitude. Learn to have an open heart. Don't be bitter. Don't be mean. Add positivity and light.

Get happy by learning to make the most of your surroundings, by being resourceful, by being creative. Learn how to identify simple pleasures that can add moments of bliss to your day.

And yes! Maybe one day you will build that corporation, marry the guy, get the girl, move to Spain and have a perfect tan.

It could happen. But until then, make the most of what you've got. Be the best person you can be in your circumstances and set the bar a bit higher.

As the day is ending here at the produce business and bikini bodies are mingling with zest at the beach, I must confess, my day here was absolutely perfect. You know why?

My husband keeps saying to me, "Thanks for being the best wife ever."

We are having a bit of our own fun during the quiet moments between customers. He just said, "Am I not merciful?"

"What?" I ask him.

"'Am I not merciful?' What movie is that from?" he asks again with a smile.

"Wait!"—I stick my hand up in the air—"I know, it's...*Gladiator*."

"Yes!"

And the story goes on, as Jared Leto sings in Thirty Seconds to Mars.

In the depths of winter, I finally learned that within me there lay an invincible summer.
~ Albert Camus

Good actions give strength to ourselves and inspire good action in others.
~ Plato

Chapter 5

Interview—with Legendary Free-Range Snowboarder, Jeremy Jones

Sometimes we need to find those already living their dreams and look to them for inspiration. We may look at ourselves in the mirror and not see the person we hope to be. There might be a sense of doubt, a feeling that what we want may seem selfish and just not important enough to this world. When I need to find inspiration, I have drawn strength and inspired my thoughts by having role models—someone I have termed a Soul Icon. This is a person who is walking their path and living their passion. They share their insurmountable goal and happiness with others. In my book, I interview individuals who share these qualities. They have passion in their eyes, that smile of knowing what it feels like to be on the other side of their dreams. They have faced uncertainty and challenging times and overcome fear and obstacles in their way. They have forged ahead with their dreams. Each person is from a different walk of life with a unique perspective from their eyes. For the Soul Icon in the 'Live' section, I must say I did somersaults (metaphorically of course!) when I finally found out I would get to interview Jeremy Jones for my book.

Jeremy Jones is a professional snowboarder, known for big mountain freeriding. He rides trails down mountains no others (or very few) have ever seen. He also hikes up to the top—more like climbs up to the top—so he can ski down high-elevation mountains. Forget helicopter rides. He is a mountain climber, too.

I found out about Jeremy Jones last year when my husband and I watched his movie, *Further*, an exquisite documentary that is visually breathtaking about his journey freeriding down mountain peaks all over the world. I must say, I was truly inspired by his passion. What I loved most was his quest for solitude and peace within the quiet spaces of the mountains. In order to achieve this, many days of hiking and climbing add up to his journey in order to achieve that ride down the mountain.

Here is my interview with Jeremy Jones on how he *lives* his passion:

You have climbed mountains and skied down mountains all over the world and are known as the athlete that pioneered big mountain riding as a snowboarder. You are an example to many as someone fearless and soulful because of your distinct life-choice to follow your heart and become a professional snowboarder. Where did your nerve come from to believe you could achieve such heights and live your passion? Could you pinpoint at what age you knew this was your destiny?

Jeremy Jones: By the time I was 10 I knew I would live in the mountains. By high school it was clear that one way or another I was going to set up my life so I could snowboard every day. All my focus was on being a pro snowboarder. I had no backup plan but if it did not work out I knew I would find another way. By 20 I knew that any chance of a 'normal' life was off the table. I had experienced the highest of highs and there was no way I was walking away from that for the security of a normal lifestyle.

In your movie, *Further*, I was blown away by the beauty of the snow, the peaks and sheer remote locations that looked like pieces of heaven. You discuss 'getting away from it all' and why that is so important to you. Why do you think that can be so beneficial to someone and their inner peace? What is it like to be on the top of one of the highest peaks in the

world that you just climbed with your own hands and snowboard? What is that moment of silence you feel before you descend the mountain?

Jeremy Jones: That moment is really just the cherry on top of the sundae. The guts of it are the journey it takes to get to the summit. It is a special feeling standing on top of a mountain I have put so much mental and physical energy towards. The mountain tops are a sacred place and give me a great perspective. Without that journey the summit has much less meaning. However, the summit is really the halfway point because I still need to get down the mountain. So the real celebration comes at the bottom of the mountain.

What advice could you give someone that is considering quitting their day job and is afraid to make the leap into doing what they love? If they are not talented enough to pursue a living doing what they love full time, would you consider a hobby the next best option for them to try?

Jeremy Jones: Do not make reckless decisions. If this great change keeps calling at you and you cannot get it out of your thoughts then start plotting your next move with much care and thought. When you have vetted your idea as best as possible there will be a moment when all that is left to do is jump off that cliff. Make that leap with every ounce of energy you have. Life is too short not to go for your dream. If on further review you realize that quitting your job is not the smartest idea then a hobby is a great alternative.

How has being immersed in the rugged mountain snow peaks and the beauty of nature been beneficial to the quality of life you experience each week? Do you think that's something beneficial to all—even those who work a hectic schedule and for those who have cosmopolitan city lifestyles?

Jeremy Jones: My life seems to get more and more hectic every year with raising kids, running a business, etc. This is why unplugging has become so important. It is a mental recharge that gives me a perspective on life that I cannot get any other way. Even disconnecting for a little bit every day helps. All my serious life-decisions have been made outside when I am disconnected. The more serious a decision, the longer I like to unplug. *Vacation response works! Use it!*

Do you see a direct correlation in your level of peace and happiness by having the courage to live your dream daily and being an example to younger snowboarders following in your footsteps? How has your lifestyle been affected with your family and friends because of choosing to do what you love?

Jeremy Jones: Following your passion is the most important thing in life. I am surrounded by people who have made these choices. It is like we all forged our way down a road full of pitfalls and have made it to this beautiful utopia at the end of the road full of people living life to their fullest. My kids are growing up surrounded by many different types of people with jobs ranging from lawyers, builders, moviemakers, stockbrokers, professional snowboarders, etc. But they all live an impassioned life.

What is your next big adventure? What would your last words of encouragement be to someone sitting on the fence of their dreams because they are only seeing the current circumstances that surround them?

Jeremy Jones: Right now I am focused on some closer-to-home backyard adventures. I love the simplicity of hopping in my car, driving to a mountain range I have never been, hiking in with everything I need for a few days and exploring the range on my snowboard. My advice to people on the fence: life is a gift, life is now.

'Life is now' is a line I don't want to forget. So take words of advice: find out what lights your heart on fire. Jeremy Jones is climbing mountains, and skiing down them all over the world. He found his passion and made his dreams happen with intense focus and practice. I must admit that I was quite thrilled to interview him regarding how he continues to dream and pursue his passion. He is my first Soul Icon as an example of someone LIVING their passion. Could this be you, too? Make it happen. Get busy, and don't be your own self-defeatist. Get out there and *live*.

Definition of 'bucket list':

A list of things that one has not done before but wants to do before dying.
~ Merriam Webster Dictionary

People talk about this 'bucket list': "I need to go to this country, I need to skydive." Whereas I need to think as much as I can, to feel as much as I can, to be conscious and observe and understand me and the people around me as much as I can.
~ Amy Tan, *New York Times* Bestselling Author

Chapter 6

Have a Bucket List

I used to think bucket lists added to the thought of focusing on death and dying. I did not like the thought of that. I found that after much discovery and learning the true definition of 'bucket list', it can be many things to many people. As you can see from the gifted writer Amy Tan, it has a different meaning to her than exactly what it could be to you. The idea of making a list at first seemed contrived, silly and just not worth my time. I also thought that it was more geared for a later age…which could be true for some, too.

But what I have found from developing my own personalized 'Bucket List' mid-life during my early forties is…that it's FUN! Why? *If you make time to make wishes, write them down and believe in them, the chances are you will work toward making them come true.* And if that just happens to be skydiving…do it! Make your list and think about it. Cultivate it. Germinate it. Believe in your life as a grand adventure. It's yours to create. So definitely take time for that bucket list, which I used to misunderstand. It's good to have a little fun and to dream.

One of my favorite philosophers of all time was a British man named James Allen at the turn of the 20th century. He was a pioneer of the Self-Help Movement and wrote one of my favorite succinct philosophy books, *As A Man Thinketh*.

I'll never forget the first time I read his book back in 1998. It was Thanksgiving weekend and I was going through a mild depression due to mononucleosis. I felt horribly run down, all at the ripe age of 27. So I turned to my favorite section at Barnes and Noble and plucked up this little yellow book that looked vintage and resembled a mini-size coffee-table book. I took it with me that Thanksgiving weekend. I remember feeling absolutely numb to the beauty of the ocean, the clean streets and the posh hotel full of fancy soaps and deep bathtub in my hotel room in Santa Barbara. But luckily I had this little book with me, which truly did wonders for my soul.

I lay in the hotel bed and fervently gobbled up the pages of this book. It sank in like medicine can after we have been run down and our bodies react quickly to it. I started to enjoy the sunshine and acknowledge the beauty of my loved ones around me that weekend. The surf and sand of Santa Barbara began to shimmer across the horizon.

But to this day, I have a clear vision and feeling of the first time I read this next passage. Early in the morning, the day after Turkey Day, I drank my coffee and turned the pages of the book to chapter six. When I read the first line, I sat up in bed like a cannon might shoot someone out of it at the circus. I flung upright with buoyancy when I read the next line:

Dreamers are the saviors of the world.

My God.

I had a chance!

If anyone knows after recovering from being ill or from a disease, fighting your way back is maybe the hardest part of all. Even though my illness was more associated with a kissing disease, my immune system had been thoroughly shot and my mind and body were weak in spirit, too. Reading this simple passage was like receiving a Vitamin B shot to my soul. As a constant dreamer and thinker of things to come, I realized I could discover more in life.

James Allen's next few lines fit with the 'Bucket List Theory' and why we should foster dreams:

He who cherishes a beautiful vision, a lofty ideal in his heart, will one day realize it. Columbus cherished a vision of another world, and he discovered it. Copernicus fostered the vision of a multiplicity of worlds and a wider universe and he revealed it. Buddha beheld a vision of a spiritual world of stainless beauty and of perfect peace and he entered into it. Cherish your visions. Cherish your ideals. Cherish the music that stirs your heart, for out of them will grow all delightful conditions, all heavenly environment; of these, if you remain true to them, your world will be at last built.

So the question is: do you believe this statement? I do! I had never been so inspired by one sentence in my life as I was that one weekend when my soul so needed to read and learn those words. If I had to say there might be a moment—a turning point—I could link my recovery of believing in dreams and thinking lofty ideals to be that weekend. I knew that James Allen had discovered and shared a monumental secret about life. He revealed it not just to me, but all of us!

So are you ready to make your bucket list? Are you ready to carve out and build the rest of your remaining days on this planet to a vision that could require something more of you as a person, as a friend, a wife, a mother, a lover, a companion? Are you ready to envision a list that moves your spirit to wake up with more enthusiasm because you know just what it takes to make your dreams become a reality or something you can do? Let's do one right now together.

The Bucket List

- Make a list of places you might want to visit in your lifetime.
- Make a short list of accomplishments that would make your heart sing if you could accomplish them.
- Make a list of internal needs and desires that can improve your daily well-being.
- Make a list of any philanthropic things that you would like

to be part of or contribute to, which could add more love to your heart because of the 'giving factor.'
- Top 'fun thing' to do you have always wanted to do. Something that could make you extraordinarily happy.
- *Now pick and choose just a few from each list and fine-tune it to fit what could be your Ultimate Bucket List.*

Here is an example of some things on my List:

- Take a trip to Captiva Island, Florida. I would love to go there and write for a week or even a month. *A Gift from the Sea*, by Anne Morrow Lindbergh, was written there in a small beach bungalow.
- Visit St Rita at Cascia, Italy. She is my favorite saint and has given me much comfort in time of need by keeping her medal close to my heart.
- Take more time to learn how to paint and paint more Impressionist paintings.
- Contribute time and energy to saving animals that need homes, whether that be through fostering, sharing information or adoption.
- Go to Puerto Vallarta, stay at this little Bed and Breakfast where the owners rescue stray dogs from the street. I want to shake their hands, feed the dogs and hang out in their hammock above their infinity pool and watch the sun set, while the doggies play nearby.
- Go to the town of Aracataca in Columbia. Why? This is the fictionalized town of Macondo that Gabriel Marquez made famous in *One Hundred Years of Solitude*, one of my favorite novels.
- Go to French Town, New Jersey and stay in the quaint Bed and Breakfast I follow on Facebook. Then visit the antique shop, Two Buttons. Elizabeth Gilbert's husband is the owner and it looks truly magical!

- Be more loving. Smile more each day and show more compassion and empathy to all. Beat out the judgment and find compassion.
- Become a foster for Dobermans or start a non-profit Doberman rescue. My red Doberman, Fortune, has been such new inspiration and joy in my world, I hope someday I can help someone else find and save a Doberman like my dog, Fortune.

Just now, even as I wrote those down and shared them with you, I found a certain enjoyment by thinking about them. Life is meant to be lived, experienced, and you are meant to be a Live Love Soul each day. In order to achieve that, it requires a little time, dreaming and action to get us on our way. So the next time someone mentions their bucket list, give them a little smile of reassurance. Because this life is ours to create. We can take the steps to make our future happen. Bucket list? Yes, I now have one! I think James Allen would approve.

PS: Sometimes we don't get to experience all of our wishes and dreams. But thinking of them might be just enough to help us get through one more day. Start dreaming and visualizing your next adventure. You can make it happen. And if you don't get to mark them off your list, don't worry. Sometimes there is just pure joy in dreaming and thinking of tomorrow.

Motivation is the fuel necessary to keep the human engine running.
~ Zig Ziglar

Chapter 7

How to Stay Motivated

I am a big believer in caffeine. I remember during my twenties I had confided to a friend that whenever I was down, I just brewed myself a big pot of coffee and instantly felt a relief from that gray moment surrounding my soul. Caffeine motivates me. I like the taste of it. I like to make it. I have it etched in the memory of my heart when I grew up on my childhood farm in Missouri. Guess what? We didn't have the Internet or a smartphone or even cable television. But we did have a coffee maker that always had a pot of coffee ready to go. My family still loves to make coffee and sit around the table—whether that be early morning, afternoon, or late into the evening. We know that with a good cup of coffee in hand, anything is possible.

Hence the thousands of Starbucks, the coffee shops, the artists who used their caffeine to kick-start their day. I recently gave up coffee for a few days and just drank some green tea. Later in the week I confided to my husband that I had been a little down and not feeling motivated like normal. (I try to keep it at a cup a day. And the good news is there are lots of supporting articles on the power of coffee and why you should be drinking it. But do consult your doctor and remember: everything in moderation.)

"Baby, we need to buy you some coffee."

He brought home some Yuban and made me a fresh cup. I instantly perked up, found my groove and remembered that, for me, coffee is one of those motivators that makes my life tick.

This chapter isn't about coffee, but it's the first example to you of what works for me and motivates my soul and body. A little ritual that helps keep me sane, alert and with it. I know. You may be one of those anti-coffee gurus that believes in only eating vegan and staying away from caffeine. Hey, if that is your motivator, that's more power to you. Exactly my point.

What motivates you or lifts your spirits? Do you have a 'go-to' daily ritual that can zap your soul into *happy mode* when you need a lift? Don't worry, I only drink one cup in the morning, and on grand occasions I will indulge in an Americano. But at least I have one tiny key, one thing I know can help me get up out of bed and make my day start off with an alert mind ready to tackle what may come my way.

So you're not a coffee drinker. Make your fruit smoothie or stick to your hot tea. But do find something that can help boost your motivation for the day. As Zig Ziglar stated, "Motivation is the fuel necessary to keep the human engine running." It is important to define things, techniques and ways that can help us stay motivated so we don't run out of fuel.

When we lose our motivation—I can add myself as an example of this. I can give the description of my long teal underwear top and my leopard pajamas that comfort my motivation-less nights with a TV clicker and sloppy up-do bun with a good choice of skinny ice-cream bars handy. I have to admit, it's kind of fun to take a break from being motivated. Everyone needs a pajama day or two. Just make sure it doesn't turn into a long stretch of make-up-less days that have you just scrolling your social networking feeds for the next update status.

Another simple motivator is wearing my Nike lycra running pants. I am pretty much guaranteed to work out if those things make it onto my body. I feel like I can clean the house, walk the dog and run four miles, all in a span of an hour or so. It usually takes two hours or so for all of that. But that's how it makes me *feel*. I ditched my running shorts for these guys and my only comparison could maybe be what it feels like for a Superhero to put on their Superhero outfit. Run out and buy a pair. You won't regret it.

Stay Motivated and Connected to Life

This is essential to our well-being and our daily happiness. So in this chapter you need to uncover what you think could help you feel more inspired. How can you learn how to motivate yourself in order to improve your mood and schedule? Maybe it's working a bit harder at your current career. Maybe you are a stay-at-home mom and you struggle with keeping the house clean because you already do so much. How do we find inner motivation when a flat-line is beating across our spirit? You need to find your key 'jump-start' motivators that get you going.

What does a pack of motivational supplies look like?

- Friends that want to take you higher. Yes, first of all, start with your relationships. Do you have a negative crew hanging out around you? It may be some time for internal relationship weeding (this is discussed in another chapter).
- Follow or subscribe to a motivational person. Maybe it's your favorite author or it could even be a motivational public personality. My favorite right now is Les Brown. Reading his daily posts on a social networking site can sometimes be that one 'kick-in-the-butt' I needed.
- Exercise more. Yes, that's right. Get your body moving early morning and watch the rest of your day fall into perfect position because you made time 'for your health' and for yourself. Endorphins will motivate you naturally.
- Keep little sticky notes on your mirror or on your refrigerator of uplifting literature to keep you smiling. Maybe it's even a Bible verse. "I can do all things through Jesus Christ who strengthens me" (Philippians 4:13) has motivated my brain and heart through many of my days.
- What sits next to your bedside table? Keep a few books there that are tangible—even if you are a Nook or Kindle

reader—that you can feel and touch in your hands. Mark up the pages. Underline the passages. Follow some sound advice. Elizabeth Gilbert and Michiko Rolek have been my great motivators next to my bed.

- Have a go-to ritual that you can fall back on in a crisis or a hard day. Besides my early morning coffee and bird-watching hour, I also know if I head to my favorite second-hand bookstore, even just for 10 minutes, my soul will elevate out of my sneakers and a slight smile will find my lips again.
- Have some fun! How do you do that? Act a bit silly in the car. You know, sing out loud. Sing off key, sing like a wannabe *American Idol* winner, and who cares if someone in the next car is looking? Be-pop your head like that guy in *A Night at the Roxbury*. Create some fun each day and motivation will surely follow.

Exercise: Now is the time to take that quiet moment you have created with your yoga mat. Grab your pen and journal and try to discover little things you can do each day to keep you motivated.

That's my list. It's not too long. It's not too short and it's not just about caffeine. It's about waking up and fighting for a better day by staying motivated on my feet. So make time to create an environment that is more positive and enriching. Trust me, life is a battle. It's not always easy. So one of the little tricks is to keep yourself motivated within your own schedule so you feel some joy along the way. We must create these moments. No one else can get busy for us. So find your motivators and use them! And yes, have some fun, too. Don't forget to be-pop your head the next time you are driving in your car, and do play Abba. I heard they are making a comeback.

You have to find something that you love enough to be able to take risks, jump over the hurdles and break through the brick walls that are always going to be placed in front of you. If you don't have that kind of feeling for what you are doing, you'll stop at the first giant hurdle.

~ George Lucas

Chapter 8

Breaking through the Walls

In 1998, I had come to the end of a few decent years as an actress and model in Los Angeles. My new life was emerging around me as I began to tap into my inner desires. During this period I worked with a life coach who helped me go deeper within to discover what direction I wanted to go with my life. Could I dare say it? Could it be...*a writer*? Writing is a lofty-sounding career where it's either very well respected or the folks just think you are some dreamer writing a string of words together. Yes, there was Ernest Hemingway and John Steinbeck and Pearl S. Buck...and now welcome to our generation of coffee-table writers sitting there with their laptop, bagel and a latte, feeling rather intellectual about themselves. The distance between the great and the wannabes may equal the distance between the Earth and the moon. So when you figure it out in your mind that this is what you want to do, trust me, there was a metaphorical row of domino walls ready to fall when I went about pursuing my heart's desire.

Well, one night I had to prove to myself this writing thing, you know. I had at that point written some poetry, kept a journal and had furtively done my morning pages when I read Julie Cameron's *The Artist's Way*. I had attended some workshops and creative writing classes, but there hadn't been that body of work that I could own that made me feel like "Yes, indeed! This is where I belong." Sometimes before we shift our foundations and our livelihood we need to prove it to ourselves first that we are worth that and we can do and accomplish our heart's desire.

How I broke through my first writing wall:
1. I set a goal. I made a decision after speaking to my acting

agents who said they were willing to submit a play (I had written one act and it was well received). They would be willing to submit it to the HBO Workspace to see if it would be accepted as a showcase.

2. That night I had been out at a coffee diner on Sunset Boulevard at 1 a.m., sharing my ideas on philosophy and life with some other friends; it was then when I realized it was time to head home and to face that fear and just jump through and go for it. So I left them abruptly, drove home and then began a surge of typing late into the wee hours of the morning. I remember watching the sun rise through the windows. I remember feeling an exuberant feeling of accomplishing this mission—this thing that I so desperately wanted, but had been running from. I then took that week, cleaned up my three-act play, gave it a title and waited to see what they thought...

Oh, the fear of being nothing.

It loomed. It did. And for one week, I drove around in my big black pick-up truck waiting for that answer if...*I was good enough to continue.* Looking back now, I realize that whether or not my agents decided my writing material was strong enough, I would have kept writing. But at least I had the *nerve* to break a barrier—a wall—that had been holding me back at this point in pursuing my passion.

The answer came back from my agents that they would indeed submit my material. I then went on to produce, showcase, direct my three-act play a few months later. The HBO Workspace invited new artists and writers 'by invitation only' to share their work and utilize their facility. I remember telling a good friend when I left Hollywood, out of all my bookings and jobs, that invitation and showcase night was the biggest and most satisfying thrill nestled among these rolling hills of Mulholland Drive.

Soon after that, I signed up for an extension writers' program at UCLA. I remember those nights fondly. I carried big books and wore long skirts. I hung out with other aspiring writers and real writers. I took my notepads and went to work with others consumed with the same love of writing. This was before the full-blown computer and Internet invasion. I remember others discussing if they needed a computer really to be a writer when they already had a typewriter or word processor. I remember the others looking at me and summing up my bright blonde hair with wide eyes as a need for acceptance, and turning away…just slightly enough where I always felt like 'the pretty girl that was trying to be taken seriously.'

I remember one teacher telling me my books were "OK if you didn't mind having it at the airport in the book section" and that I wasn't literary in her sense of the word. I remember walking out of there completely thrilled. I wasn't aiming for a Pulitzer—I just wanted to be a writer. I wasn't her genre, but she could see me fitting in somewhere. I remember another teacher telling me my words were "lovely and I emoted well on page, which was a gift not everyone had." I remember reading *In Cold Blood* with the rest of the class and feeling really with it and good about myself for the first time in years. Although my face, blonde hair and appearance looked anything but literary, I had never been happier traipsing through the dark winter evenings on the UCLA campus to attend those late evening classes. I might just have to rank that up with the play.

Now you might be thinking the next thing that happened is— yes, I became published and I found an agent and the world opened up for me since I broke through the wall with my writing desires.

No.

That was only the first one. Life comes in a series of chapters. We must be willing to flow with the changes. You might need to tote your inner passion with you. Instead, I moved down to sunny San Diego with my husband and was pregnant, too. Soon, I hopped into motherhood, wifehood and almost forgot about my own dreams. It can be hard to do that when there is so much busyness of life with motherhood and new beginnings.

That little dream of writing stayed with me though. So I began to read as many books as I could. I went to Barnes and Noble when I could with my newborn baby to find exciting fiction books to read.

I called upon my therapist, Tess Hightower in Los Angeles, when I hit writer's block again and asked for guidance. I couldn't seem to find a way to break that next wall that was attempting to hold me back. Reading was all I could manage to do with the early morning mom hours and such.

Tess inspired me to set a small goal of writing seven pages a week. She calculated that I could finish this novel I had begun at UCLA in under one year if I just stuck to this simple writing program. I then went to an extension writing course in San Diego on 'how to finish a novel' to gain courage at this task. All of the baby steps led to me finding my way back to that magical lit-up blue-lighted computer after nursing and feeding my baby. I would wear the same little pair of pajamas, drink one glass of chocolate soy milk before I began, and then slipped into my fictional world and those fabulous characters. And at the end of the week, I would send my seven pages to Tess. Those pages added up. I finished my book.

I drove to San Clemente and had a bowl of clams and a glass of wine to celebrate my mini-achievement: one more time to break through the wall.

This story continues. I will continue piece by piece through each section with you how I stayed on point and kept writing when another wall threatened to hold me back.

Walls—How Do You Break Them?

What I have shared with you are mini-examples of the walls of fear that I broke through in order to achieve a dream and find my passion. As you can see with my own journey, sometimes what we want takes time and patience to make our dreams materialize and come true.

What we don't always realize, when we want something from within, we must remember that this is *our own desire, our own destiny to create*. No one else can do it for you. Some may expect overnight success. They may think that what they want is unattainable. But I am here to tell you:

Follow the greats. Become inspired. Find someone who can inspire your mind to help you achieve your dreams.

My journey as a writer happened in tiny steps, the right ones that led to bigger doors opening with time:

- publishing stories in the newspaper
- maintaining a writing schedule each day
- writing covered featured stories for magazines and online websites looking for copy
- being a newspaper columnist

Becoming a writer over the years felt like *bliss* to my soul. And of course, this doesn't mean it wasn't work. What we love can become 'work,' too. I did everything, such as write a short novella, a long fiction novel, and enter a few writing contests. Eventually after solid years of writing for newspapers and magazines, my husband suggested that I focus on non-fiction since that was where I had found my voice as a published writer. I opened up my heart and took his advice. So my question to you is:

What wall do you need to break through in order to attain your dream?

- Take a few moments one weekend and make some quiet time so you can organize your thoughts on pen and paper.

Maybe even in your little smartphone yellow notepad section. I would suggest manually writing it out in a notebook, maybe a tiny one that slips into your bag or your back pocket so you can carry your dream with you.

- Write down what it is you want to do. Be patient with your dream.

- Devise a realistic plan made up of smaller goals that can help you attain your dream. When I say be realistic, I mean be realistic.

- Don't expect to become an overnight success. And most of those you think were overnight successes weren't either. One of my favorite writers, Elizabeth Gilbert, expressed to her readers that she "was an overnight success if you counted the twenty years" it took to get there. So be prepared to go for the distance. If this is your passion, then you won't care because you will enjoy carving out the steps it takes to make your dream a reality. And with passion comes hard work. Just because it is something you love to do, does not imply that some nitty-gritty work won't be involved, too. So don't be afraid to get your hands dirty.

- Talk up your dreams. And be bold! Don't share your dream with just anyone. You must protect it so it can grow, receive light, and bloom with proper care. Not everyone will think your dream sounds attainable. And then there will be some of those mean people out there who will tell you or hint that you are an idiot for even trying. *Let their insensitive words of doubt fuel your dream... Just ignore them.*

- Take action. What does this mean? Yes, do something physical and implement your goal into a true reality. You can't just go around in dreamland and keep your head in the clouds. You must take proper action to make your dream see the dawning of a new day where you are actually living it, bit by bit.

- *Pray!* I am a big believer in prayer. Prayer enables us to have faith in the unknown and to materialize what we cannot see. Prayers fight fears and help us break through the walls trying to stop us. So be humble. Swallow that pride and get down on your knees and pray your heart out. Pray for your dream.

- Let go of the past and past failures. Start over each day with the thought that today you can take small measures to attain your wishes and dreams.

Breaking through the wall of fear that threatens to defeat us can be done with hard work and tenacity. So dig in. Think BIG! And don't let the unknown 'wall of fear' stop you from advancing forward. Don't give up. Don't give in, and make sure to keep having fun. Why? Because life can be short. So wake up smiling and just *go for what your heart desires*. It may take a lifetime to carve that out, but for now, little bits of joy will be singing for your soul's inner happiness.

PS: I often hear many say they aren't doing what they love and their job is not their passion. This does not mean you cannot still find a vivacious life and make other dreams happen. Just having a 'job' in this day and age is a gift. So don't quit your day job because you hate it. Show gratitude and respect to your boss. Be grateful for your pay check. When the time is right, you may find the right opportunity to find a new job that will settle well with your soul. We aren't all destined to be Van Gogh. So don't discount your normal life as nothing. Take pride each day in what you do. Smile. Be grateful and try harder to be a person that exemplifies gratitude. You never know, that 'job' you dislike might become a great source of joy someday soon. Life is always full of miracles right under our nose. We just need to tune into a higher frequency to recognize them.

The measure of intelligence is the ability to change.
~ Albert Einstein

Stay committed to your decisions, but stay flexible in your approach.
~ Tony Robbins

Chapter 9

Be Flexible. Life Can Change on a Dime

I had it all planned that day. I had made the reservation. Packed my bag with my computer, two favorite inspirational books and my personal journal so I could handwrite my thoughts in the tranquility of the woods. There was a little cabin in Idyllwild, California waiting for me with a key reserved for me. For two weeks I thought about it. I reminisced. I saw myself in the little cabin in the woods reflecting, thinking, writing and just taking in the solitude of nature all to myself. *This was the plan.* I had been there before with my husband for our special anniversary trip only two months earlier. So I knew what I was doing. I had been there before. I've got this handled.

That day, I scrubbed and mopped the floors at the house at lightning speed. I walked our Doberman. I vacuumed our carpets. I even watered our plants in our tiny yard located in the quaint beach town of Cardiff-by-the-Sea. I had this day mapped out as the perfect destination that would soothe my soul for weeks to come. This would be my first writing trip alone, away from my family. You know, allowing me to bank in those 10,000 words you read about on the Internet that some writers are able to do. I have had some long days like that. But during this stretch of time, I had not seen a number like that in my tiny Word document corner in a while.

Right before I headed out of town on my mountain journey to seclusion and a carefree writing space, I stopped by to see my husband. We programmed in the directions to Idyllwild. Then I set off on my little journey. The drive I had done before. It was a cinch. I just waited for the little voice on my smartphone to guide me up the mountain.

Well, two hours later I had not arrived. I was sitting in stop-

and-go traffic in a little town called Hemet, just below my destination. For some reason the GPS took my journey on a different
route. I was not prepared for this. A bit of fear welled up in my
stomach. You know, that debilitating kind that can warn you are
in danger.

Then I started my mountain ascent up the road to my destination of bliss and reprieve. There I would feel welcomed by the
solitude of need in my soul. The part that needs to retreat from
the noise of family life, the routines, the meals, the same schedule
week after week. A departure from even just walking my dog.
Sometimes it's important to switch it up.

As I viewed the hairpin curves and the direct mountain
descent just a few feet away from the road, my heart lurched
again with fear. I had not taken this road before. Was I on the
right road? I pulled off on a mountainside passing section where
cars that are driving at a slower speed can be kind enough to let
the seasoned mountain drivers pass. I checked my GPS.

Oh, shoot. There was a glitch. It hit a section where the directions turned off, but I could still see the location of where I was,
I thought. Or was that actually right?

Confusion set in. Then fear. Then uncertainty. I looked over
the mountain edge and found the sense of adventure leap
forward with a plunge. This was not what I had been expecting.
I had it planned with an easy journey set forth with the perfect
destination. After all, I needed to get away…right?

Instead, I was lost on a windy mountain road with the loss of
my bearings and the sense of fear clutching my gut. I had to
admit it to myself—I needed help. I called my husband.

He pulled up the map and informed me that he thought I had
passed my turn-off and I was actually driving down the
mountain into Palm Springs. So I turned around and headed
back. Except where was the turn-off?

Where was it? The little cabin of retreat was waiting for me…

Some plans laid out ahead of us seem certain because we have made them. But there may be a different outcome awaiting us when we had our hopes up for something else. We must be able to shift with the changes and be flexible.

You might have guessed by now—I never made it to the cabin. I never made it that day. As I drove down the mountain my car began to shake and I thought for sure I might be having one of those scary 'woman moments' where I was vulnerable out in the wilderness with nothing but a pepper spray and a car that quit on me too. Fear came up so fast again that I said a tiny prayer in my head: "God, let me get home, please. Let me make it back."

My husband then called; I managed to 'hand-free answer the phone.' He informed me that I was actually almost there and that I just needed to drive back up the mountain. He had been wrong about driving into the Palm Springs destination. "Just turn around, baby, you are almost there," he had said in a reassuring voice.

But after the car shaking and those hairpin turns on the mountain highway, I had had enough adventure for one day. I managed to drive back to San Diego safely without breaking down.

Of course once I made it down the mountain, my car was fine. Luckily, owners of the little cabin were very understanding and let me rebook my trip for another time.

That day I drove home after driving for almost five hours to nowhere. I managed to drive up a mountain and turn around and drive back home. I felt like such a failure for some reason. You know. Here I am a grown woman and I can't even do a trip properly on my own. I didn't cry any tears of pity but I wanted to. I think the fact I was so relieved just to make it home in one piece outweighed my disappointment.

Home never looked better. My Doberman looked like the answer to safety. My husband's arms felt so warm and inviting. I discovered the value of my own personal world from an unexpected journey gone wrong.

Sometimes in life we make plans. We design them and build dreams around them. We count on them. However, life can take us a different direction when we least expect it. The trick is to relax, be kind to our souls and allow ourselves to make mistakes and not make life always such a 'life-and-death matter.' (Although that mountain 6000-foot drop was pretty steep!)

My little journey instead revealed that my wonderful life looked pretty amazing. Surely I could hit my word count again in the privacy and safety of my own home.

I did not have that little cabin mountain escape nestled among pine trees. My plans were changed by unforeseen mistakes and I had to reroute my destination. Finding our bliss is not always attached to a vacation. It can be right under our nose.

That particular day, I learned to take my own advice. I found the journey of five hours, which led me back to home, also took me to a deeper place inside my soul. The cabin in the woods will be there for another time. And if I don't get to make my great mountain escape for my writer's retreat ever, even though that little two-day trip never happened, I had so much fun thinking about it and imagining my journey.

Dreams take us to places we want to go. And sometimes they take us deeper into our own self-discovery. Make sure that you allow for some pitfalls, side streets and unexpected roads you didn't plan on taking. Because when you least expect it, your journey could turn out differently. Just don't let it knock you off your center. Why? Life is always a mystery still waiting to be discovered. So don't get too attached to the outcome.

One mishap or unplanned road might take you to your heart's desire.

For it says that no matter how hard the world pushes against me, within me, there is something stronger—something better—pushing right back.
~ Albert Camus

If you never try, you'll never know what you're worth.
~ Chris Martin

Chapter 10

Why *Trying* Is Something You Should Do

Sometimes in life you just have to jazz it up a bit. You gotta get creative. You need to find a new rhythm. Explore new territory that you have never seen. Dare to broaden your horizons—with life being an endless 'to-do' list of family, work and getting up to do it all over again. (Please note that even if you are a world traveler or a single who wants to stay single without children, life can sneak up on you and become *routine*.)

So this is a chapter dedicated to you, dear reader, on how you can find something new and exciting that your soul hasn't experienced. Yes. It's time to sweat, get uncomfortable and try something new.

Isn't that the worst? Feeling like there is something missing but you can't quite squeeze out of your comfort zone because:

1. You may think you are too old to try something new.
2. You don't have the brain capacity to learn how to be creative.
3. You are too lazy. Why try anything new when I can just continue to 'scroll' my phone, watch new and exciting movies, or read another book on Kindle?
4. You just think that your view is fantastic and you've done everything. Wrong. There is still something new to discover. Knitting? Hot yoga? Have you tried ballroom dancing, painting, a book club, a workout group? Trust me, there is something new out there waiting for you to discover... What?

The New You

Maybe the best way to help you understand this chapter is to share with you how I am pushing my own limits, too. And this isn't an easy share. I would rather roll over and tell you I am an excellent runner. Unfortunately, after hitting runner's burn-out around 40, I had hung up my running shoes and began walking with short breezy runs in between. A real runner knows this is definitely not running. So for three years of being off my running feet, I had to learn the hard way of how to come back and learn something new all over again.

My Story—and Why 'Try' Is a Cool Word

Well, honestly I didn't think I would be sharing this story in this book. I thought that it would come after, when I could put a better 'spin' on it as they say in Hollywood. However, I have come to realize over the last three months that this little struggle of mine is something monumental in everyone's life.

A mistake many of us make is we just operate on 'go.' We continue to get up, do the same thing and produce the same type of productivity in our lives.
If it isn't broken why fix it?

But who wants to live a life with that quote hanging in their minds? Who wants to just get by? I know I do on occasion because it is easier. It's easier to do what we think we can instead of challenge ourselves beyond our own familiar limits.

So imagine me on my 43rd birthday this year, reading *The Shining* by Stephen King, and lying in my bed watching the clouds linger by as life continued on my easy path of existence. I took my advice and decided to cross one off the Bucket List. It's a big one for me.

Run a Marathon

So as the world crept into the stillness of my room in between the 'REDRUM' and green hedges that became alive at the hotel (the maze was added in the movie—no maze anywhere in the book—

and trust me, the live bushes were scarier), I took a moment to sign up for my first marathon before the year 2014 ends. Then I went back to *The Shining*, my coffee, and had no idea of the new chain of events that were about to occur from making this one decision.

One month later, I started running again. Well, maybe I should say breathing heavily and finding a few good strides during a couple of miles. I must admit that it didn't look promising. This marathon loomed larger than life and I had no idea how in the world I would ever accomplish that amount of miles when even two were breaking me down into a 'sweat ball.' (I've never been one of those cute workout girls in the pink spandex outfits who look perfectly cool with their make-up on. I'm one of those 'run hard, play hard, sweat a lot' types because I'm not that cool!)

A couple of weeks into this training bit, I began to feel quite overwhelmed by these weekly miles. And let's face it, I'm not 33 anymore and running a half-marathon before was relatively easy. But a marathon?

Why had I stopped reading *The Shining* to do that Bucket List thing?

Oh yes, to challenge myself. Fabulous.

Well, I could keep going on. I could tell you at one point how I called my mom and broke down into tears over the whole thing. I could tell you that I dreaded running with a passion. I would clean, read, write, anything other than do my necessary run.

But I continued to toil. I did. I got uncomfortable. I even bored my husband to death with updates on which foods worked better and how my run went minute by minute. I began reading obsessively every runner's world story I could get my hands on...but still, I had hit a WALL just trying to run, before real training even began. I had only been clocking about 10–12 miles a week, which is low mileage for running. This was me. My growing uneasy in my skin was making my mind spin with agitation, and that 'inner critic' voice was out to defeat me.

But as Jerry Maguire so aptly stated in the now famous movie, *Jerry Maguire*...you know the scene, where he just got flipped off by the kid in the hospital because the kid's dad had five concussions? So Jerry finds himself back in an unfamiliar hotel room and writes a mission statement and says in his mind of thoughts to the audience watching as the movie plays: "Breakdown, breakthrough."

So one night as I was going to bed with the lights off, and I was all snuggled in my pajamas, preparing to get up in seven hours to run, I heard a voice. Call it an angel, my higher self — whatever you feel like if it will make you interpret this better — a *voice*.

And it said, "Why are you doing this?"

Well, of course, because it's on my bucket list, right?

"Why are you doing this? Do you know? What is the point of doing this if you don't know why you are doing it?"

You see, many times in our lives we set out to achieve goals, but if we don't know the *truth* in why we *want* to achieve this goal or to attain this new thing, we can't really make progress. We don't get to go to the next level until we understand the view from where we are.

So back to me under the covers in the dark with that daunting voice in my mind asking me why I wanted to run a marathon...well, I thought about it. And it came out rather simply actually.

I LIKE RUNNING. I want to be a runner again. There it was, so simple and pure.

That pivotal moment of understanding why I had to do this, or at least try, became something new to me. I had a new spin on it. It was like a breath of fresh air. The world opened up and I saw that this was just something I love and I am trying to do it.

After this experience, yes, the *breakthrough* came. I began my mornings with my early morning run with excitement and joy. I actually stopped drinking teas and coffees halfway through the day so I could crawl into bed and go to sleep early. Before my long weekend runs, I could be found soundly asleep before 10 p.m. on a Friday night. Hey, this wasn't a glamorous existence, but I had found my stride and began loving my running shoes.

I eagerly awoke in the wee early morning darkness to make my coffee. Then I found my running shoes and I ran. I clocked it with my Runkeeper app, listened to the music and enjoyed these silent early morning runs. Slowly but surely, the miles are piling on and now I am up to 25 miles a week. Then I hit 30. This may not seem like much to an ultra-marathoner who might be reading this book. But for a middle-aged-mom who hadn't run in over three years, this was definitely my breakthrough moment.

I am such a novice runner. But guess what? I am a happy runner now. I am so excited to try this and to get out of my comfort zone and learn something new.

I may never become some athlete runner that goes out and runs a lot of races in a year, but at least I am trying to do *one new thing*. And because of this, I have had to work through some uncomfortable feelings of doubt and insecurity to achieve this level of excitement.

If you are wondering how the marathon went, it's still seven months away. I am climbing slowly to my super-long runs on the weekend with great preparation, from sports drinks planned, orange slices in little baggies, to a perfect playlist. I even have the 'Rocky' theme song dialed in, which of course may make me the biggest cheese-ball ever. But I am running with bells on in my mind.

We must remember to challenge ourselves to break rhythm. We must get all out of sync with our lives in order to discover another aspect of our soul that may have not been tapped into yet. The journey within is the most important. What have you not discovered inside of yourself yet?

Exercise: What is your list? What would you like to try to do but haven't?

- Take a little notepad, or better yet a journal, or even your smartphone notes, and write out some ideas and achievements you have always wanted to do but haven't.
- Now figure out which one could work with your current schedule. Is this something you can feasibly do without physically hurting yourself? (Be realistic with your goals.)
- Write out at least three. Then narrow down to the one that will make your heart sing and will be the one goal that can jump-start your life. Remember to ask yourself, "Why do I want to do this? Is it for the right reasons? Will this benefit my life?"
- Now choose your goal, grab your calendar and make it happen.

Regarding my own uncomfortable zone, I hope I can do it. I hope I can cross the finish line. I hope I can hit that mile 24 on the Big Hill I've read about on the course and muster up every last drop of belief and excitement in me. I hope I can. But in the meantime, I am learning more about myself. I am happy I am *trying* this.

So many times we don't TRY because we are afraid to fail. I say: TRY anyway and have fun in the process. You might discover the YOU you've always wanted to become.

So don't be down on that little word. Don't be down on what it can lead to: accomplishing your next dream. You can do and be anything you want to be with enough trying behind sweat, tears and joy. So get creative and start dreaming of something new to do.

Update: My outcome here ended up being a half marathon

instead of a full. One of the key factors in going after our dreams is sometimes we may need to modify them if what we have set out to do does not necessarily work out for us. Running a half marathon that day in Santa Barbara, California under the 80 degree sun was a big enough challenge for me. My heart sang with joy that moment as I crossed the finish line.

At one point when I had become discouraged, I thought about throwing in the towel altogether.

But then I remembered, "Be flexible in your approach," you know that great quote I share by Tony Robbins? And it resonated with me. I found out I could use my bib number for a half marathon instead. I shook off those feelings of failure and I still showed up for what my body could actually do...well. It's important to remember, if a goal is too big and you find yourself not hitting it yet, you may need to take baby steps and modify your approach.

I am so glad though that I set out the path for the big one because that journey of training and what I learned in those early morning hours last year while the world was sleeping was worth it. The best part is I had so much fun training.

So don't beat yourself up or become discouraged if you might need to modify your dreams. Remember to keep going and celebrate the mini-victories. If you don't no one else will.

Theodore Roosevelt once said:

"It is hard to fail, but worse never to have tried to succeed."

So what's next? This year I am immersed in Yoga! Remember, keep it interesting, switch it up and keep dreaming a new dream so you can have more fun each day on your journey.

We are the hero of our own story.
~ Mary McCarthy

Chapter 11

The Ladder of Life—Reach Up and Grab On

Life can be disappointing. We don't always get what we want or what we need, as that famous song promises us. We can turn down a road we did not foresee. Wait! This wasn't part of my plan. This was not what I had predicted or wanted. Life can be...*hard*.

Yes, I've been there, too. I will share with you that one of my hardest periods would be when I went through a divorce in my early thirties. Talk about feeling like a...what? *A big fat failure.* This was not what I had envisioned and I didn't see this one coming. A single, divorced mom sounded like a person I did not know. I had been the 'actress,' the 'model,' the 'writer,' but 'single and divorced mom'? Not what I had envisioned as a child.

So imagine me in my little apartment sitting on the side of a valley in Carmel Valley, Southern California, sitting on a patio alone with a 2-year-old baby...now what? Oh, I took to meditating. I took to running 5 miles a day six days a week. I focused my energy on 'being the best mom I could be.' I went to Barnes and Noble and thumbed through many self-help books, discovered numerology as a hobby and had some fun moments with my friends. I prayed. I lit a candle on my bathroom floor with my hands on the Bible and laid out my fears silently to God and my soul. But the fear would not subside. The feeling would not abate. The fear was stuck in my throat each day. I felt constricted by my new limitless life without surrounding walls that defined my future. I felt...*afraid*.

Luckily for me, I have a dad with much wisdom. I remember calling him up and telling him about my fear. Tears were there. I felt utterly down. Then he asked me this sort of silly question:

"Are you afraid the 'bogeyman' is gonna get you?"

"No," I answered.

"Well then, what?" he retorted.

"I don't know, Dad. I just don't know what I am afraid of anymore."

"Don't be silly. Just keep on. Reach up and grab the next bar on the ladder. All you have to do is reach up and grab it."

"I think I can do that… Okay, Dad."

Well, that made a lot of sense to me. This vision of the ladder and grabbing one more bar. I could see that clearly. I could imagine successfully grabbing that bar and pulling myself up to the next step. This mental image was something that was a 'go-to' thought that centered my 'little voice' inside of me doubting myself and my thoughts. I held onto that each day. I saw that moment, reached up, and felt success in my mind because I was still climbing the ladder of life at least in my mind.

We know that many athletes use visualization to help them achieve consistent and optimal performance by harnessing their thoughts, seeing what they want to happen, and then go about the many hours of hard work of training to prove their vision to be 'true.'

So if you are at a scary time in your life right now, apply a metaphor that can firmly be planted in your head that makes sense. This might help you overcome your fears, too.

Matthew McConaughey just won his first Oscar this year (2014). His acceptance speech truly inspired me and I admired his attitude toward his journey and thought process. He recounted how someone had asked him, "Who is your hero, Matthew?" He responded, "Me in 10 years." That may sound a little narcissistic, but what he was feeding his mind was that his future self was the man he wanted to become. He became the 'hero of his own story' like Mary McCarthy suggested in that quote that should resonate with your soul. His positive visualization and dreaming of being better than who he was, and what he wanted to become, kept his heart and mind motivated to 'keep reaching for the next bar,' and not give up or become complacent with his achievement. He had more to conquer, more to become, more to be. He had a vision and it was of himself—being a bit greater than where he was at a younger age.

You might say, "Oh yeah, easy for him. He is a movie star." But remember, he was just a kid from Texas without any ties to Hollywood with a clear vision and a dream. He worked through his own dark moments and kept grabbing the next bar on the ladder without fail.

You can do the same. So this chapter is to remind you, if you are struggling or feeling down, to cultivate and believe in something more of yourself. Believe that you are the hero of your own story. You may feel alone. You may be lonely. But take your mind and imagine the angels surrounding you when you go forth; imagine your big strides of tomorrow and know that the darkest hour will break. The hurt and anguish *can* fade.

I remember in my mid-thirties, I called my parents to express, "Maybe I'm not meant to find The One." Somehow, after thinking that and realizing that if that were to be, I could still manage to have a fantastic life on my own, I stopped looking for The One and got busy following my life, my daily moments, and found much happiness by letting go of circumstances that felt overwhelming and defeating. I began to focus on what I could achieve, and do *each day*, instead of worrying about things out of my control. I found my confidence by 'grabbing a mental image in my mind' of pulling myself up to the next level, and that made me feel good about myself again.

I just read a fantastic line in *The Gunslinger* by Stephen King. The Gunslinger meets a young man in the desert and gives the man some simple instructions to help this guy deal with his fears and plight: "Don't feel sorry for yourself. Make do."

This is true in life, too. 'Making do' doesn't sound like much fun, but it's plausible and helps us get through one more day.

85

Sometimes that's the key to pulling out of the darkness and into the light. The light is there, just on the other side.

So don't give up! Don't give in! Find your momentum. Say 'no' to the little voice that is hard to turn off in our minds. Do the opposite. Plant a firm vision of what you would like your world to become and see it clearly each day. Imagine it. Dream it. Feel it. Feel it deep inside your bones, in your heart. Say, "Thank you! This is mine. I will get there."

For me, my little vision of writing happened with many baby steps of hard work and not reaching for some unrealistic goal. I focused on 'making do' with my own realistic surroundings and what I could achieve now. I found a job at a newspaper when my son was in kindergarten. My foot in the door was through the advertising department. But that soon led to writing press-release stories for my clients and printed by-lines in the paper. I began to build my résumé. I rebuilt my world by taking my dad's simple advice and 'grabbing the next bar' on the ladder in life.

I didn't shoot too high. I grabbed what was attainable and in reach.

The girl on the floor in her bathroom meditating over a Bible and flickering candle made it out of the scary dark times and found her footing because she held on for one more day. One more day might just be your answer. *So don't give up.* Grab a mental metaphor that inspires you to push through to your next day.

What to Do to Make It through the Hard Times

Exercise: Mat time! Grab the journal and pen. It's time to make a list and write positive affirmations.

- Work on silencing the negative voice in your mind. Instead firmly plant a positive visual that makes sense to your line of thinking and is something that you can understand and apply each day that will help silence the negative thoughts.

- Enlist a mentor. This could be a therapist or life coach. Sometimes we need guidance outside of our circle. They could be a counselor at church...someone you can trust and who can help you find your momentum again.
- Ask yourself, "What am I afraid of? What is on the other side of my fear?" Uncover what that fear is and how you can conquer it within you. Make do. Look around your current set of circumstances and discover tiny goals that you can achieve that will help you chip away at the fear that has paralyzed you. Take action. Don't just think it. You must do the thing you fear and put it to rest.
- Hang in there. Don't just self-obsess. Find a hobby. I took up painting during this time and it was just a good diversion from wondering if I would ever work my way out of the apartment stuck on the Valley overlooking a dried-up molehill. *Divert the fear. Develop a hobby.*

Get busy

Discover something new. What was my discovery? The philosophy of numbers based on the father of mathematics, Pythagoras. What fun I had uncovering the meanings behind a number and figuring out someone else's life path!

Pray! Never underestimate the power of an honest, heartfelt prayer.

Talk up yourself. Shift the small voice into a positive voice, one that pokes fun at your fears and enlightens your mind to find a smile during the hardships.

Imagine yourself in the future. The YOU you want to become. Believe it and take those realistic baby steps to hitting the big strides. Life is a mystery. So carve out yours for yourself.

Now take time to write about what fears come up for you and what actions you are going to take to defeat them.

Reach up and grab on! Why?

What is around the corner could be just what you are waiting for on your journey! This life is worth making your very own. And guess what? "The Bogeyman" isn't gonna get you. And you might even find your smile and have some fun again real soon. So hold on, make do and become the hero of your own story. You can do it! I believe in you. And if you are wondering…five years later in my life I met a really wonderful man. I didn't end up in the tiny apartment alone near the dusty valley. I had to wait for a bit for his arrival. But guess what?

I got busy living and having fun. The Bogeyman never did catch me. I think I figured out a way to outrun him. You can, too.

Bogeyman is "an imaginary evil spirit, referred to typically frighten children." If this seems too silly, insert the word FEAR. I do believe there is a Clint Black country music song about him, too.

The miracle isn't that I finished. The miracle is that I had the courage to start.

~ John Bingham

Chapter 12

Interview—with Dr Jason Karp on the Benefits of Exercise and Running

Everyone has their thing that helps them find their peace and solitude. If you don't, I hope these pages inside this book will motivate you to discover what that is for you. For me, as you can see from this book, having activities, daily planning and actions that I take have been my biggest resource to discover 'organic daily happiness.' It's not out there waiting to be a feeling. You can bring on happiness by striving to do small tasks and simple actions to improve your mood. And if this can be true, why not try?

I have been a runner during different periods of my life. There was even a time when I used to run around the Lake Hollywood dam five days a week and enjoy the view of the Hollywood sign. I would listen to my cassette tape and would listen to Madonna. And if life couldn't be a little more surreal than that, I would actually pass her running around the dam with bleached blonde cornrows. Madonna and her bodyguard, too. You could say back then, I just took little things like that for granted. (Celebrities are all over Los Angeles. And soon you realize they are just folks like us. And good for Madonna for staying in rock-solid stellar shape.)

So here I am now over the age of 40. I have turned to running once again to find my groove. Running longer distances and at fast paces can be challenging. So I have once again turned on my headset that is now connected to my smartphone and I am listening to Thirty Seconds to Mars fueling my 4-mile run early in the morning.

One important factor on this journey to finding happiness is making your physical health a priority. Maybe you aren't into running. But it might be easier than you think. You don't have to run races to exercise. You might just need some tennis shoes and workout clothes.

I am thrilled to interview Dr Jason Karp. He just happens to be one of those locals that I was lucky enough to feature in my column every so often for their running group on Mondays, running under the glorious eucalyptus trees on the trails in Rancho Santa Fe.

Dr Jason Karp is also a marathoner, author and fitness coach who helps runners reach their goals. His book, *Marathons for Dummies*, was front row and center in a Boston bookstore during that week of the most famous marathon in the world (plus many other running books). I was thrilled when he agreed to be interviewed on the benefits of exercise and running.

Here is my interview with Dr Jason Karp on the benefits of running:

What advice would you give someone who has never run before, but is thinking about becoming a 'fitness runner'?

Dr Jason Karp: Just literally walk out your front door and start running. It's really that simple. If you can't run for long, then mix walking and running. All humans inherently can run. It's in our DNA.

I have been a runner during different periods in my life. Each time I was consistent as a runner, I can link that time to being in a stable and prolific creative state for my mind. I find that when I have been a real 'runner' a lot of my ideas for writing came to me. Why is that? Why does running tap into something deeper in our mind? Do you feel this is true?

Dr Jason Karp: Yes, it's very true. Running has many effects on us, including effects on the brain and the ability to think. A number of studies have shown that exercise improves fluid intelligence, which includes problem-solving ability, memory, learning, and pattern recognition. Improvements in cognitive function with exercise are even more observable as people age. Exercise enhances the connections between pre-existing nerve cells in the brain and enhances the formation and survival of new nerve cells. Running also puts us in a state of relaxation, which fosters creativity.

On someone's quest to find happiness in their life, how interlinked is exercise to this equation? If someone isn't exercising regularly, what advice could you give them to motivate them into at least setting smaller goals to get them going?

Dr Jason Karp: Exercise is strongly linked to happiness because when you exercise you feel good and when you feel good, you carry yourself in a different way. You feel better about yourself, and how you feel about yourself influences how you interact with others. For someone who isn't exercising, the best advice I can offer is to find something that makes them feel good and set a small goal that they can work toward. Having a goal provides direction and motivation to attain it.

What has running done to improve your life, your attitude and your sense of well-being? How did you fall in love with running?

Dr Jason Karp: It all started with a race once around the track in sixth grade. Even before that, during the Presidential Physical Fitness Tests we did in elementary school, I found out that I was faster than most of the other kids. But my love started with running track in middle school. It felt good to see

how fast I could run. Running has improved my life in more ways than I can articulate. It has made me a better person. It has taught me how to be patient. It has taught me how to win and how to lose. When I'm really fit, I feel better about myself and I walk around with a lot more confidence.

What are the immediate perks someone can expect from becoming a fitness runner on the treadmill and outside in their neighborhood? Start slow and then add miles?

Dr Jason Karp: There are many perks, including better fitness, a nicer-looking body, and much better health. Start slow, and over time as your body adapts and responds to the stimulus, add miles and then add intensity.

I have read that running can help lower risk of getting breast cancer for women because it lowers estrogen levels. What other health benefits can someone expect if they become a runner, even later in their life?

Dr Jason Karp: There are many health benefits from running, including decreased risk of cardiovascular disease, increased bone density, decreased percentage of body fat, increased metabolic profile due to increased oxygen delivery to and use by muscles, decreased risk of diabetes due to an enhanced responsiveness of cells to insulin, decreased risk of certain types of cancer, increases in cognitive function, enhanced self-image, decreased blood pressure, decreased cholesterol, and decreased risk of mortality from all causes.

Any last departing words you would like to add regarding why you have devoted your life to running as a doctor, author and trainer? Why is this your passion?

Dr Jason Karp: This question would take a long time to answer, and I'm not even entirely sure if I know the correct answer myself. Running is so much a part of who I am that I don't question it anymore. I suppose part of the answer is that running has given me a chance to explore who I am and who I want to be. It challenges me in a way that few other things do. When my mother was in the hospital for the last two weeks of her life, I had to run every day before going to the hospital each morning. Running gave me the strength to cope with her dying. So I could be stronger for me and for her. What else can give someone that kind of strength and resolve? I suppose that's why I have devoted my life to it.

I hope that inspired you to consider buying a brand-new pair of sneakers! Don't be just one of those who watch on the sidelines. Get busy and find out why running might just be the thing your life could use to infuse your soul with inspiration and excitement. You don't have to run a marathon. You can just run in your neighborhood or at the gym. Don't miss out on what many people all over the world already know. Running can take you mentally higher and also help you stay in shape at any period of your life. So rock on and...what? RUN!

Part Two—Love

Spread love everywhere you go. Let no one ever come to you without leaving happier.
~ Mother Teresa

Be curious, not judgmental.
~ Walt Whitman

Chapter 13

Non Judgment. Melt Your Heart from Judging by Inserting These Two Words

I grew up in a Southern Baptist church in the Bible Belt of the Midwest. I remember that I wanted to take it all in, understand the meaning of Christ, God, and this life. I wanted to get it right. You know that feeling when you want to get it right and not wrong? What exactly is that feeling? I had to find that out, too.

When I left my small town in Missouri to live in San Francisco, you could say culture shock was an understatement. From driving around on a two-lane dirt road, I found myself searching for blades of grass in an architecturally gorgeous concrete jungle. I was in awe of San Francisco. The food, the folks, the buses, the BART (Bay Area Rapid Transit)... The Golden Gate looked like the most magnificent sight I had ever seen. I even wrote a poem about it in Los Angeles a few years later that honestly didn't make sense to anyone in the coffee shop that day as I stood up at the open-mike night, except for me. I was trying to convey that significance of the curves, the concrete, the bridge and a dream...I am getting off track. Let's get back to those Baptists I grew up with in the Midwest and a young woman on the beginning of her journey in San Francisco.

When Two Worlds Collide

I soon noticed a theme with those I met when they asked me, "Where are you from?"

"Missouri." (I soon stopped saying the small town or even the nearest town near where I was raised because no one there had an inkling of anything that existed in a fly-over state.)

"Wow, thank God you got out of there!"

Yes, this was normally the response, and then some. Plus

about how backward those who lived there were. Pretty rude, huh? I felt rather slighted by these new folks. You know, how could they say such things so blatantly? What about Southern manners? *You never insult someone's roots.*

But then, guess what? I would go back over the holidays and experience that same prejudiced stance. Except this time it was from those I grew up with in a small town. "They're just a bunch of weirdos out there, ain't they?" (Well, no. But they think you are a hillbilly, too.)

I soon found out this would be an ongoing theme in my life. Trying to figure out *what* was right and *who* was right. I mean, if those liberals in San Francisco were so liberal and negative about people where I grew up, then was it really any different from the ignorant and conservative thoughts I had heard from my Missouri folks? So the question was: where did I fit in? And what was right? After all, life was a vapor. I am here for a short time; I want to make sure my thoughts are on the right track.

This middle ground of existing between these two worlds revealed to me the importance of one word:

Tolerance

Definition: *The ability or willingness to tolerate something, in particular the existence of opinions or behavior that one does not necessarily agree with.*

Due to this polar opposite theme that never truly changed with each year I lived in California, I quickly learned to keep my thoughts to myself, and what I really thought—my opinion—was just that. Keep the peace. This became my mission.

So I endured many years of listening to this back-and-forth banter about the Midwest and why California folks are stuck up and weird. I lived each year wondering: why are we so harsh? Why can't we just learn to accept and not be *judgmental*? During this period, I began to practice something I still practice today. This mind exercise helps me a great deal. I feel more peace in my heart. I also find more happiness because my thoughts are shut down from that one inclination we all have, which is to judge others.

When I see someone that rubs me the wrong way, instead of beginning that internal dialogue in my mind about "What an idiot, what are they thinking? Your underwear is hanging out! Maybe you want to do something about it," I quickly insert these two words: *non judgment*. I say that in my mind and it stops my internal dialogue, helping my moral compass to shut off with those two exact words:

Non Judgment

What does it mean?

Non: Not doing; not involved with; 'non-aggression.'

Judgment: The act or process of judging; the formation of an opinion after consideration or deliberation.

Think of this as more like being non-judgmental in an instant. Try saying "non judgment" in your mind and see if it helps you to eliminate that negativity cycle of wanting to judge others.

What happens when I do this?

Well, I don't use up my thoughts with negative thoughts. I tune out devaluing someone else with a judgment that could be based on the wrong circumstance. We do not know what happened to this person today. We don't know why the homeless person is homeless. We don't know why that driver just flipped us off at the stop sign. So don't react. Don't judge. Teach your mind to be calm and insert these two powerful words.

Learn how to tap out the judgment part of your mind in your daily thoughts.

What can I do instead with my thoughts? Channel a nice prayer toward the stranger. Shoot one right at them! Zing them with well-wishes. Don't spoil your time with hazardous thoughts that can spoil your mind. Stop them in their tracks. Learn to make space for peace and beauty. Shut out that critical voice that wants to be so critical of others. You have the power to silence it!

This has helped me find so much solace and peace over the years. You know, we are each just trying to survive. We are each just trying to survive our own journey. So be nice and try not to *be right*. Send love from your thoughts. Your powerful thinking toward others in a gentle and peaceful manner benefits you the most. And also them. You are signaling a positive energy to them. You are sending them blessings versus judgment and belittling thoughts. Send love! Maybe there is a chance they can feel that. You might be shifting their day with the power of love.

Looking back as a child in the Baptist church and learning my Bible verses, I so wanted to get life right. What I learned with age is that 'the right life' does not exist. Why? Because we are all so different. Life is a mystery. There are not always answers to what may burden our souls. Knowing this, there should be only love and human compassion toward others. So find tolerance. Build a light and put a damper on that inner critical voice that wants to rule the world.

Remember these two powerful words: *non judgment*. Let those two definitions do their work and give your mind a break from the idle chit-chatter.

After all, life is but a vapor...so don't waste it with mean, critical thoughts.

Your inner voice is the voice of divinity. To hear it, we need to be in solitude, even in crowded places.
~ AR Rahman

I fear the day that technology will surpass our human interaction.
~ Albert Einstein

Chapter 14

Take 'Mini-Me' Breaks and Discover the Gift of Solitude

Recently I have stepped away from my social networks. All of them. Just for a bit, you know. I took a few minutes on my smartphone and deleted all of my major apps that I find myself scrolling daily for updates: Pinterest, Facebook, and Twitter. I know. Truly a chapter on technology?

Well, absolutely. I think now more than ever we as individuals need to harness our self-control and take mini-breaks from these fabulous apps and gadgets that keep us so entertained…or is it distracted?

Where Is the Soul?

This was originally my first working title when the concept of the book emerged. I constantly look around and see heads down and eyes glued to technology. I am sure you do, too. There have been a few poignant documentaries capturing this recent problem in society.

And yes, I am guilty, too!

That's why I take mini-breaks. It's good to give your mind a rest from others' status updates, the latest-trending news topics, and which pin on Pinterest is too hard to pass up.

Our soul is just like a garden. It needs tending. It needs watering, love and care…and most of all our soul needs *our* attention. If you keep your mind preoccupied without allowing it time to breathe into a place of quiet rest, how can your mind find time to think of anything original without what you are thinking being triggered by what you are reading?

Quiet time is the essence of the small space we need to step into to find out our purpose. If you stay checked out of your daily schedule by keeping your mind occupied, you inadvertently are neglecting your soul.

What do you need to do? Make time for yourself, too. Step away from technology. Take 'Mini-Me' breaks

Schedule time for yourself. Delete your favorite apps and make space for YOU. Get to know yourself. Listen to your thoughts. Direct them into a happier place with positive thoughts and self-affirmations. Don't just be on automatic in this life. Learn to show up each day for yourself. Learn to be present and not just distracted and busy. If this is difficult for you to do, try to do this for a few hours on a designated day.

I find that when I take these mini-breaks, my soul feels *happier*. I read more. I rest better and take time to do little joyful moments for just me. Of course, I think, "What am I missing on my friends' feeds? I love them so, I need to know." But soon that feeling dissolves. And I am back to just me, my thoughts, and can feel the quiet space that allows my soul to breathe freely.

I am tapping into that special place where miracles can happen. My mind is quiet. I feel more calm and grounded, like for example last night:

I did my stretches, while reading a classic, *The Old Man and the Sea*. I sat there in the quietness of my bedroom as the moonlight lit up my outside terrace. I contemplated this relationship of a little boy and and an old fisherman setting their casts deep out into the ocean. I found out about their morning schedule. The rising early and getting the fishing gear, the bait and two coffees with other fishermen in the morning darkness when the world was still asleep. The old man and the boy would sit together drinking their coffees in condensed-milk tins, reflecting upon the day to come. Would the Old Man be lucky today?

These private moments to myself just felt like a big warm blanket comforting my soul.

Why? The world was quiet. I was in harmony with my thoughts. I continued to do my yoga stretches, as I read for about 20 minutes or so. The importance of that 'Mini-Me' time added so much more clarity to my thinking. Such peace surrounded me in this mini-me break.

Because of this time, it added a new thought and meaning to my night. I had recently started running again. And part of this journey has led me to reading runners' blogs on their experiences. So what was next? Just a new little place in this world for me to write my thoughts out about my running experiences. This was a good way to harness my thoughts. I felt as if I had designed a piece of my soul with laser-like focus. I worked for a good two hours on my blog, choosing colors and carefully placing my first post out there for the runner community to read. How wonderful to do a little something for me other than pinning a few pins on Pinterest and scrolling my social network feeds. This energy consisted of designing, creating and writing something that reflected my inner life and thoughts.

So taking a 'Mini-Me' break has added much joy into my schedule again. I must admit I can easily run amuck, too, with all of these fun apps. Who doesn't love searching for their favorite quote on Pinterest? Who doesn't like seeing what their friends are up to? We all do. But we must force ourselves to disconnect that plug so we can discover what our soul may be craving.

What you need to do to begin your 'Mini-Me' breaks:

Be honest with yourself and figure out a time when you can take a break. Maybe the weekend is better? Or maybe the weekdays. You figure it out. Figure out what works for you. Start with two days. And if you can eventually do a week break, take that.

Okay, so now what?

- Take a few moments and sit on your floor. If you have a yoga mat, lay that out and sit there. Make a private space just for you. Sit comfortably. If you want to add stretches, do that, too.

- Get a handy notepad or spend a few extra dollars on a beautiful journal. You will need to have a pen handy, too.
- Now take a few moments to breathe. Take five deep breaths. Breathe deeply into the core area of your body, almost as if you are filling your stomach with air. Then release this deep breath with a little slight "Ahh" sound and count to one. Do just five simple breaths to arrive in a more quiet and centered place.
- See what is coming up. What do you love? What do you miss? Are you sad, or are you angry? Observe the silence and the feelings.
- Write down what comes up. Write down what you are feeling. Why do this? It's important to process our thoughts and feelings and to be in touch with our emotions. Don't let your emotions run your life. Let them become more like fluid water that can roll in and out without disturbing your 'center.'

Now ask yourself:

- "What do I love?"
- "Does something seem to be missing?"
- "How can I add more vitality and joy in my week by doing something more of what I love?"

I hope this exercise has helped you uncover a hobby you have forgotten that you love to do. Maybe you used to be a reader or have a thing for collecting music and studying lyrics. Maybe you are an early morning bird-watcher. Maybe your heart misses hanging out with loved ones who are no longer in your life. If feelings of loneliness come up, it might be time for you to step out of your *boxed-in world of technology*.

Take a brisk walk in your neighborhood. You could even join a church, a monthly book club, or just join a gym or the local YMCA to place yourself into a situation where you are out and about with *real people*. Don't just hibernate. Don't be alone too much. Our soul needs to connect with others so we can express and share this precious journey we are given together.

Try to Do 'Mini-Me' Breaks At Least Once a Week

If you are dealing with a lot of untapped anger or sadness, it might be wise to seek counseling or a support group.

So get creative and learn to take time away from that iPad you so love carrying about in your purse. Learn to be silent with yourself so you don't miss out on a golden opportunity to get to enjoy your very best friend on this earth that needs your attention. Who?

YOU! In order to build new dreams, we must first visualize them and create them in our mind. If we are too busy, there is no room for that silent voice from our soul that is waiting to guide us to a new and exciting adventure. Learn to love yourself. This minor adjustment could help you in more ways than one. It might lead to discoveries, all because you took time to tap out of the tech world that can zap our brains dead if we don't watch it.

So don't wait for the love of your life to do it for you. Don't wait for the right set of circumstances. You must get busy now making moments for solitude so you can uncover *your voice of distinction*, guiding you to what brings your soul delight.

What is my newest love? My anonymous running blog that inspires me to keep running! I am so happy to discover this new dream existing within me. Without my mini-technology break this last week, I might have missed that yearning. So get busy deleting your apps. Take a break and spend more time with YOU. I promise you, you won't regret it.

Meaning of white roses:
Purity, innocence; acceptance; unconditional love; feminine or passive energy

Encourage, lift and strengthen one another. For the positive energy spread to one will be felt by us all. For we are connected, one and all.
~ Deborah Day

Chapter 15

Extend the White Rose of Love and What Would *Harvey* Do?

I recently had my first book published. It has been a much-loved adventure. A much-loved endeavor, but most of all a much-loved connecting with new friends and authors through social networks. I find it quite exhilarating to receive support and love across the net these days. Life can be tough. So when you receive more love, doesn't that help, too?

I don't want to beat around the real subject though. I want to address why you must always:

Extend the white rose to your friends and loved ones when they have worked for something. Even if it's a crossword puzzle. Extend the rose and give them your blessing.

White roses can symbolize unity, honor and friendship. This is more of a metaphor for you to imagine—yes, just like the olive branch! This is what you need to remember to do during those important moments in your loved one's life. Extend the white rose and give them that all-important seal of approval.

You might not want to. You might think that their achievement is rather inane, silly or trite. You may smirk to yourself in the corner of your room at their pride in the new 'tiny' victory in their life. Maybe it's a huge one to them. But to you...well, please!

Get Ready to Wipe Away Your 'Inner Meanie'!

Definition of 'meanie': *a mean or small-minded person*

Is that who you want to be? No. Reach for the white rose.

Extend your approval. Even if you aren't so sure what someone's measly accomplishment is, don't diss it. Why? Life is tough enough without your closest circle chipping away at your accomplishments. So don't be the person who throws the thought of insecurity on your friend's minor victory. Even if you think it's a minor *nothing*.

Extend the white rose. Show love. Life is tough. So spread the love. You will feel better in the long run, too.

Sometimes we can't see someone's achievements because we think we know them too well. You know, "We must be honest with our loved ones and tell them what we think." Operative word: *we/you*. After all, being honest is sharing the *truth* of our *thoughts*. They know every little flaw. They see the light, the dark and what's between. Maybe that's why when success comes into the picture, friendships can suddenly end. So ask yourself: are you ready to give up your Inner Meanie? Lord knows I am! I work on silencing that Inner Meanie, too.

So, why can't we just be happy for our friend's successes and their joys? It's time to place our egos in check. Do your own internal work and extend the 'white rose' to your friend looking for a pat on the back. Especially if they value your opinion or if you are their mentor! By all means, squash those negative critical words and support them.

If you aren't a hundred percent behind their achievement, you don't have to say "I loved it" or "Fantastic!" You can find a more diplomatic way to share your support. Spread joy and experience the afterglow of giving your friend that 'pat on the back' they were hoping for with their grand achievement. Give them the spotlight. Let them shine. Just remember, your turn could be next.

Life Is a Series of Complicated Matters Really

Did you know a suicide is happening in America every 16 seconds and every 40 seconds around the world? *So tread on your words lightly.* Hold that tongue. Think before you speak. Why? Your opinion doesn't really matter except to you. So get out that white metaphorical rose and start giving already, would you?

I will share with you now, before this chapter ends, an example of a fictional character who nails this metaphor and meaning:

Harvey
(Created by playwright Mary Chase)

Elwood P. Dowd is the main character in *Harvey*. Here is a tiny synopsis: He believes he can see a 6 ft 6 inch rabbit. His family thinks he is insane. So his family checks him into a mental institution where he begins to receive therapy from the psychiatrist. But in a surprising and heartwarming plot twist, the doctor can see the rabbit, too. He asks him in so many words, "How have you been able to put up with everyone thinking you are crazy when you know the rabbit is real?"

Here is Harvey's heartwarming response: "Years ago my mother used to say to me, she'd say, 'In this world, Elwood, you must be'—she always called me Elwood—'in this world, Elwood, you must be oh so smart or oh so pleasant.' Well, for years I was smart. I recommend pleasant. You may quote me."

The simple fact is we don't need to educate others in the ways of the world or take measures to dash their successes. Life is cruel enough without our harsh words of honesty, which could be painful to the person we love. So make sure you are being careful with your inner circle. Make sure you aren't unintentionally dashing someone's dreams with your opinion. You could be breaking their heart and ruining a friendship.

Is your opinion worth risking a friendship?

So think before you speak. Hold your tongue before you speak *your* truth. Not everyone needs to know your nitty-gritty thoughts. So, yes! Be pleasant instead of being right. Tread lightly with your words. Don't be a person that's breaking another's heart or is shattering a dream. Ask yourself: what would Harvey do? I think you will find you're the answer.

To love oneself is the beginning of a lifelong romance.
~ Oscar Wilde

This self-love is the instrument of our preservation; it resembles the provision for the perpetuity of mankind: it is necessary, it is dear to us, it gives us pleasure, and we must conceal it.
~ Voltaire

Chapter 16

Cultivate More Self-Love

I remember thinking as a child, "Jesus loves me." How wonderful, I used to think as a child. However, I also remember thinking at such an early age, "I don't want to focus on me." Isn't that *selfish thinking*? The words 'self' and 'me' conjure up an immediate thought of thinking only of one's self. I have discovered, through my own trials and errors, that *self-love* trumps the rest. It's like that safety vest under your seat on the airplane. It's also the air supply dangling above you when you are in flight. Without it, you will not survive the crash.

What I have learned over the years about the importance of self-love and why this should be at the top of your Love List:

Self-love runs deeper than your biological clock. It runs deeper than the changes in seasons. Self-love may be the only warm blanket you can find when hard times hit and your friends desert you. Self-love should be your best friend. Self-love is about cultivating an inner life with your 'soul' and learning about what makes you happy and what doesn't. Self-love isn't boring. It's the most important love you can learn.

Self-love will come in handy when you choose your friends.

Self-love will come in handy when you find a life partner.

Self-love will come in handy when you sleep alone at night in a queen-size bed for a few years, while you are living out there on your own, discovering yourself and big dreams on the journey. Self-love talks positively to you at night. It tells you you are enough. When the lights are out and that fear breaks through the silence and threatens to steal your self-confidence, self-love tells fear to take a hike and to leave.

Self-love will tell you, if you are having a bad day, "Don't worry, there is a new day tomorrow, and one bad day does not equal a lifetime." Self-love will help you reinvent wishes and dreams. Self-love will seek out a mentor or a teacher who can help you facilitate what you need.

Self-love will help you dream...BIGGER!

Self-love blankets your heart from hurt and disappointment. It reminds you that better things are yet to come. Self-love will reach down to the deepest of your core and beg you to:

GET UP! FIGHT! And believe in yourself and your life and your dreams.

Self-love will bring you into a scary place of lonely times. It may weed out shallow friends. Self-love will ask YOU to strive for a better future and a better you.

Self-love will examine your food, your drinks and your exercise routine. Do you have a hobby? *"What is your hobby?"* self-love will scream! You'd better come up with one or self-love won't get off your shoulder until you do.

Self-love believes in the ultimate You. The best of your potential. Self-love is connected to your higher conscience, your angels and your future that you cannot feel or see. Your self-love has the third all-knowing eye that is trying to guide you to a place where you belong.

So what is the most important love you can develop in this world? Self-love.

This is your inner voice, your friend, your safety net of love you can count on. Without self-love, there cannot be true compassion, gratitude or blessings.

God wants us to love our 'inner selves'—our *soul*—and to examine who and what we are and why we are necessary to this moment.

So don't skim out on the most important love. Develop it.

Fight for it. Teach yourself to *love you*. Speak kind words. Say and repeat affirmations. Read about how to develop it. Find a spiritual teacher.

Join a support group of caring and loving individuals who will help you connect to your inner and most important love of all that you need. Go out on a limb and discover how you can go deeper and brighter to make your self-love so great and so wide, you can withstand anything.

Your soul is in need of the greatest love of all. Self-love. Learn how to love yourself and watch your world fall into the proper pieces that you've been searching for to add to that lost pathway you could not find.

So let's get busy and learn how we can love ourselves more:

It's time to roll out your yoga mat or that pretty pink towel that works just as well. Now grab your pen and your journal and a Bible (or whatever book you feel can help you find peace).

Also, do you have a timer on your smartphone? Use that, too. Set it for 5 minutes and get ready to sit quietly with your inner you and speak only *kind* messages.

- Lie down on the mat with your back on the mat and your hands resting on your stomach.
- Now imagine feeling love and the feeling of warmth, like the sunshine filling your breathing as you breathe deeply, in and out.
- Think a positive affirmation here. *You are beautiful. You are special. You are here for a purpose. I love you. The most inner you.*
- "I can do all things through Jesus Christ, who strengthens me." Say this verse, too.
- Take a few moments of silence and feel that verse and your self-affirmations.

- Now when you breathe out, take a big breath out and make an 'ahh' noise. Let go of all the hurt and pain. Imagine the hurt that you may be feeling leaving your body with that breath.

Do this exercise for the full 5 minutes.

After you have finished, write down your experience and what you feel. Then also write down your affirmations and that verse. Writing down our affirmations after we say them to ourselves in this mini-meditation can help them sink further into our consciousness.

Now I ask you to do this every day if you can. If not every day, then three to four times a week. Work on loving yourself. Work on speaking kind words to your soul.

This will be the most important love you will develop in your lifetime. You will learn to be a better friend, lover, parent, child, and even a stranger as you encounter others you may not know.

If you need more guidance on meditation and exercises, I recommend Michiko Jane Rolek's book, *Mental Fitness*, which will help you with your mini-meditations that will promote more inner self-love.

Don't be fooled into thinking that posting 'selfies' or sharing a post on the Internet is an example of self-love. Self-love is a necessary part of your soul that is ready to carry you through the hardships and negativity that you may experience in life. Self-love is ready to take over so you have an inner safety-net.

Here are some defining quotes to leave you with on the importance of self-love:

You yourself, as much as anybody in the entire universe, deserve your love and affection.
~ Buddha

A man cannot be comfortable without his own approval.
~ Mark Twain

Love yourself first and everything else falls into line. You really have to love yourself to get anything done in this world.
~ Lucille Ball

Because one believes in oneself, one doesn't try to convince others. Because one is content with oneself, one doesn't need others' approval. Because one accepts oneself, the whole world accepts him or her.
~ Lao-Tzu

Why so many quotes? You must love yourself more. You must!

So get busy learning how to love the inner you. Your world and future depend on how much self-love you possess. Your self-love can save you during the madness and frustrations on your journey. It will be your saving grace. Loving yourself will guide you to safe waters and will not fail you. So don't make the mistake I did as a child, thinking that loving myself was a selfish act. Redirect your thoughts and learn to love yourself more. Your world will improve immensely.

We are not human beings on a spiritual journey. We are spiritual beings on a human journey.
~ Stephen Covey

Chapter 17

Interview—with #1 Bestselling Author from Ireland, Mary Elizabeth Coen

Do you believe a book can find you? I do. Last year a series of circumstances brought a book to me from across the wide Atlantic Ocean. Through this book I have connected with the most insightful, gorgeous author I now have the privilege of corresponding with as a beloved penpal of sorts. Mary Elizabeth Coen is the #1 bestselling author of *Love and the Goddess*, a special fiction book about one woman's journey in self-discovery, love and rebuilding her life after a divorce. Funny, deep and an exciting read, I devoured the pages on my yellow sofa in my front room with great glee. I remember standing in line at the post office to receive a book from Ireland. I had no idea that this would soon set my life on a new course of friendship, warmth and love. That's why when synchronicities occur we must take advantage of the blessing we are receiving. My blessing was connecting with Mary. I am so impressed with her spirit and desire to go deeper within her own soul. I was thrilled when she accepted my request to be interviewed for this book. I wanted to interview Mary, dear reader, so you can see the beauty behind intention, desires and dreams. How when someone makes their heart and soul their first priority, dreams can bloom and do. Hearts can open. Happiness can find a way of creeping in when we choose to love our self first and make our wishes and dreams a priority, as Mary shares in her interview:

Your book, *Love and the Goddess*, has been such a success in America and in Europe. What does it feel like to follow your heart, and reach for your dreams and see that literally pay off with the readers loving your writing so much?

Mary Elizabeth Coen: It has been and continues to be a wonderful journey, Machel. I wrote the novel I would like to read, with a quirky mix of travel, cookery, online dating, and inspiration. I had no idea how it would be received, so it has brought tremendous joy to get glowing reviews and emails from fans. It is a humbling experience to know I have touched readers' hearts in this manner.

How did you motivate yourself to follow through and finish your book? I find a common theme with many is that they start their goals and projects, but they don't follow through to the end of their goal. How did you keep yourself motivated and inspired to finish your book?

Mary Elizabeth Coen: Everyone is different in their approach to writing. First I figured out my idea for the book, inspired by my obsession with the triple goddess of Greek mythology. I then mapped it out, by drawing up characters and working out the central plot-line. I followed that plan for the first eleven chapters and then something wonderful happened as I found myself in the flow. The characters began to speak to me and tell me things about themselves, so of course this altered the entire course and later drafts of my book. I found this very exciting and wanted to learn more as the writing came through me. Most of all it increased my belief in the story line and gave me the inspiration to continue right to the end.

You seem to have a great support-group of friends who are 'positive energy.' How important would you say is having 'positive friends' who take you higher, like Oprah Winfrey suggested? Do you feel that has contributed to your laser-beam focus to follow your heart and pursue your dreams?

Mary Elizabeth Coen: Support from positive friends has been so vital to me, Machel, and I am honored to include you as one of my treasured inner group. Friends and family often prefer us to live a conventional life, working 9 to 5. Insecure people can be very uncomfortable with the idea of someone close to them writing, as if we are going to expose certain painful truths about them, even when writing fiction. I experienced this at a crucial stage, in advance of the launch. One person read my book and insisted that everything I wrote was autobiographical and not very flattering to her. Neither accusation was true but it made me concerned as to how people could possibly interpret or misinterpret what I write. I needed the support of very good friends and family members to overcome my own inner critic at a crucial time. People with healthy self-belief are not threatened by others. In fact they are generous in how they build each other up, inspire and motivate each other. I believe in the spiral of positivity, where surrendering to optimism, love and joy creates and attracts more of the same. I am very lucky to be connected to a fabulous group of women writers who exude this supportive energy.

What advice would you give to someone who feels defeated by their current circumstances? How can they change their perspective to become hopeful again, to follow their passion?

Mary Elizabeth Coen: Our perception determines how we face life, and will often be the defining difference between a successful person (sometimes with minimal talent) and a person who cannot make their mark, despite endless talent.

You really have to first believe you are magnificent in order for others to believe in you. I've worked in fashion where I saw stylists with no basic knowledge of fashion get lucrative jobs in advertising, ahead of talented designers with amazing portfolios. What defined the winners was their unerring self-belief and a lack of concern for competition. Really it stems from the manner in which each of us works what is known in quantum physics as a basic universal law: the law of attraction. I will give you an example here:

I know a very talented and beautiful young screenwriter (let's call her Pamela) who has written great scripts that have not yet been developed, despite promises from film companies. I say 'not yet' because I believe in her enormous talent. When I met Pamela a few months back, she was feeling very dejected and she had just been diagnosed with a non-life-threatening but nonetheless upsetting health condition. I suggested she start a gratitude journal and do some daily affirmations beginning with the following: "I am happy to go with the flow of life as I leave the past behind, and wonderful things happen for me every day."

Pamela objected and said she did not feel in the flow. In fact she felt her life and her health were stuck, her scripts abandoned along with broken dreams. I told her to be grateful on a daily basis for her talents and to thank the universe for the wonderful scripts she had already manifested. At this her eyes opened wide because she had lost belief in how great her work was, due to it not having arrived at the screen stage.

I urged her to see her work as very precious and something the world was waiting for. As I looked at her dressed in baggy gray clothes, I thought she might as well have Harry Potter's invisibility cloak thrown over her. I felt she was hiding from the world and I told her to make herself more visible: dress in colors and visualize herself going out into the world like the strong beautiful woman she is. I suggested she take out the latest script she had worked so hard on, and start pouring love into it for all those who may come to see and enjoy it. In order for this ritual to work, it would require her to clearly visualize and believe she could harness the power of love necessary to influence how the world would see her and the fruits of her talents. I told her to expect a miracle but to let go of any attachment as to how and when this would happen.

As I coached Pamela in this manner, she began pulling herself up to her full height instead of slouching. Her shoulders went back and she began to shine as she regained self-belief. A transformation occurred as the hermit's baggy gray sweats were replaced with colorful form-fitting clothes and she got back a spring in her step. Her health is improving and she has regained a belief in doing the very thing that makes her heart sing.

In other words, Pamela had a major shift in perception from fear and dejection to self-love. Every day ordinary people are creating miracles by working their own brand of magic. The secret formula lies within each of our hearts, and the ability to shift from fear-based thinking to trusting and loving ourselves.

What I loved about *Love and the Goddess* is Kate's self-discovery of finding what made her happy on the inside. Do you feel, just like in real life, this is 'key' to unleashing real joy by uncovering what your soul's true desires are?

Mary Elizabeth Coen: Being true to who we really are is so vital for each of us. Looking back on my life, I made a lot of choices based upon what I felt would please my parents, my husband and, believe it or not, the wrathful God of the Old Testament. As a child I was always artistic and dreamy: writing stories, drawing pictures, making perfume and even messing in the muddy outdoors.

Certain events occurred to alter my once-innocent state and I arrived at a point where I felt I needed to change who I was in order to conform. I worried about sin and the idea of evil because that was what the nuns drilled into us in 1960s

Catholic Ireland.

By suppressing my true self over many decades, I eventually became depressed and my body was in a lot of pain with fibromyalgia. My recovery began with a lengthy process of unlearning, which brought me to study various spiritual traditions and the work of Carl Jung. Little by little I began opening the door of the cage my soul was locked into. And it was finally through the pain of marriage breakdown that I came to understand the gift a broken heart can bring. My sorrow brought me back into nature and reconnected me with the joy that lived in the heart of a little girl who loved to dream, dance and create with wild abandon. I finally returned to myself.

Any last parting thoughts to the reader on what they can do to motivate and shift their circumstances if they are feeling defeated and are in a 'self-deprecating' period in their lives? How can they overcome, move on and find that spark again, based on your own experiences?

Mary Elizabeth Coen: I find meditation a great tool in assisting me to look at life through the eyes of my heart, enabling me to have love, compassion and faith in myself and others. Having suffered from crippling depression that lasted many years, I view meditation as a very precious gift. It helps me to connect with the divine spark within.

For many like me, this is part of a spiritual practice, but it is not always necessary to view it as such, since there are many different types of meditation. A good friend of mine is an atheist yet she practices mindfulness for the many benefits that accrue. For her, concentrating on the breath as it comes in and out of her body and stilling the mind all help to anchor and ground her for the day ahead. Mindfulness is wonderful for helping us live in the moment and be fully present in our lives. As a result, energy increases and whatever we are engaged in seems to require less effort as we begin to enter into the flow of life. Regular practice (if only for 15 minutes per day) leaves no room for prolonged feelings of defeatism. Believe me, it is truly miraculous.

I hope that you walked away with some powerful insights from Mary's interview. Her words of wisdom are an example to us on how we can dig in and create our dreams and wishes, too. So get busy building castles to the sky. Your future is waiting for you.

No person is your friend who demands your silence, or denies your right to grow.
~ Alice Walker

Chapter 18

Move On or Move Out If Those You Love Feed Negativity and Self-Doubt

Growing pains are...*hard*. In order to find your inner light sometimes you must dive deep within to find something more of yourself. This may mean cutting back on your social life. This may mean setting boundaries. This may mean taking the necessary steps to build a staircase to a higher ground, to a higher place that welcomes the sunlight and moments of golden colors that fill your soul.

When we set goals, consequences and reverberations will happen. Just know that in order to attain one wish sometimes you must let go of the familiar. You may need to stand in order to see above the trees, and going through the forest will require a 'shedding of skins,' so to speak. So many times we wish for something new to enter our lives but we are unwilling to let go of that new space that feels vulnerable or uncertain. Your backbone will require you to stand straighter. It could be holding you back.

In *Middle Age Beauty* I write candidly about friendships. I mention the blessings. I write about the benefits of having many friends versus just one. I still hold true to this. I believe in a community of supportive friends of either sex holding us up and helping us achieve new dreams. Make sure you have those kinds of friends in your world.

If they are the naysayers—the dream killers—the ones that leave you when a light of success shines for you, have the courage to move on!

Don't be afraid of the quiet, secret place within your heart that needs reconciliation. Don't be afraid of only hearing your own footsteps if those you love are not willing to grow with you.

Some may say, "How could you sever ties with those who have been your friends? *Aren't they your friends?*" That's the question you must analyze. You must be willing to look at your relationships carefully with an open eye. Are they positive or negative to your well-being?

Julie Cameron, the author of *The Artist's Way*, writes about this with a harsh truth. Labeled, "The Crazy Makers," these fun friends can keep you occupied with constant drama and fill your life with too much disorder. *Steer clear of them.* Find a way to wean yourself off the temporary satisfaction of hearing shallow stories about other people's lives that have nothing to do with your own.

Letting go of a personal relationship that has been with someone you have loved can be so difficult. We love them. We make exceptions. We make excuses. We give them time; we accept their actions because love does not think logically.

You must make your well-being a personal priority. Walking the road of solitude with reflective silence is not just for the monks. Being still and finding time to be with yourself above the noise of the chatter will have a payoff.

What Will Your Reward Be?

A bright tiny light that will begin to sparkle within. A new sense of pride that pricks the hairs on the back of your neck as you walk down the street, affecting your posture with grace and poise. An inner smile of knowing you did what you had to do. You let go of that one person or group that may have been negative about embracing the 'real you.'

Life is not a dress rehearsal. So reach out of your comfort zone. Stretch up across and over your current view. Dare to see a new light, a new situation with individuals who welcome you and your dreams. Don't stay small to please others. Don't hide behind the social scene just because you want to fit in. Find the courage to bolt into a new world that recognizes your special gifts and talents.

Sometimes we make friends with others because they are in our current set of circumstances. Just know that if you outgrow that relationship, that's fine. Hit the road. Discover a new mystery. What could that be? Something untapped within you that needs to be heard or expressed. Something within you that needs acceptance from the most important physical person walking this earth: YOU.

When you reach for your dreams and dare to find the next step, don't be afraid to step away from your circle. If your loved one or close friends really love you, they will wish you well and say positive words. So watch for that. Watch for the love, the comfort. Give them a chance.

With that said, *stop being a doormat*. Don't allow yourself to be beaten in with cruelty, abusive language, or ugliness like jealous or undermining behavior. Life is too short to spend it with the wrong person or a circle of friends who belittle your vision. Have the courage to move on and be alone. Have the courage to believe that you deserve better.

Okay, So Now You Are Lonely. Now What?

Pray. Read. Explore. That's right. Pray for your vision, your life that you are dreaming of, and hold fast to it always. There may not be one shred of evidence that what you are wishing for can become your own reality. You may have to work hard, chip away and work slowly for smaller goals that will help you reach your ultimate goal. Be realistic about how to go about doing what you want to happen and set action into reality.

Greatness Doesn't Wait—It Requires Action

That means if you want to be a marathon runner you have to run the miles and do the physical training to run the race. If you want to be a painter you may have to develop what your style is for a while before you see the ultimate results. The key, though, is to love NOW and know that trying for it is most of the fun. Trying to accomplish this goal that may sound absurd to someone else does not mean that you should quit and forget about it.

Stay away from the dream killers, the small talkers, the loose lips, the idle gossip that sinks ships.

Do your own internal homework and go within. Make time for a quiet space so you can find out more about who you are. This is not self-indulgence. This is about setting your life into motion and making your dreams become a reality because your vision is so strong, so real, you will not relinquish it, even when that means your friends start dropping off like flies.

Dig in. Be strong. Find courage to be without that comfortable place where you have someone to listen to you. If you really need support, find a therapist. Find a life coach who can help you find your wings.

Mark Twain said it best when he advised this:

Keep away from people who try to belittle your ambitions. Small people always do that, but the really great make you feel that you, too, can become great. When you are seeking to bring big plans to fruition, it is important with whom you regularly associate. Hang out with friends who are like-minded and who are also designing purpose-filled lives. Similarly, be that kind of a friend for your friends.

Don't be afraid to fly away. You may find what you've always been searching for. So move on, move out and don't let anyone else ever kill your spirit. Stand up for the most important person. YOU. If you don't, you may wake up 20 years later with too many regrets, upsets and a hidden anger that will forever haunt you for not being more caring for your soul. Eleanor Roosevelt also added these pearls of wisdom: "Great minds discuss ideas.

Average minds discuss events. Small minds discuss people."

Examine your relationships:

- Is someone being constantly negative about my personality or putting me down?
- Do my friends add light, or add drama and try to
  complicate my life?
- Am I allowing the wrong person to become an 'authority'
  on who I am as a person?
- Is there a toxic relationship that I may need to weed out of
  my current circumstances?
- Are you being a loving friend? Examine your own actions
  and make sure you take proper steps to mend your fence
  on your side if you have done something wrong or if you
  are adding unwanted drama and negativity to the life of
  someone you love.
- Are you being a positive source of light to others? Or are
  you being someone that rains on their parade with
  negative projections that might be originating from your
  own self-doubts?

So you may be reading this thinking, "Wow, I can't relate. I love
my friends." Then if that is the case, make sure you are taking
time to show your gratitude for your friendship. Don't take them
for granted. Those folks are hard to find. Make sure you are
adding to their light, too. Let them know you love them for their
constant support. Say thank you for their love. My favorite Icon
Audrey Hepburn said it best when she said this, "The best thing
to hold onto in life is each other." So make sure you are choosing
wisely. Get rid of the vampire suckers who steal your inner
beauty. You are better off without them.

Sleep is the best meditation.
~ The Dalai Lama

Women need solitude in order to find again the true essence of themselves.
~ Anne Morrow Lindbergh

When you're young, you don't realize the sacrifices that people are making for you.
~ Bobby Orr

Chapter 19

The Three S's for Helping You Find More Love and Happiness

My sister often tells the story of when we all lived on the farm back in Missouri. I always find it cute when I hear it. "When we were kids, Machel would just get up and put herself to bed without anyone telling her to go to sleep when she was a little girl, which always amazed me." That might not be the exact quote but something to that extent.

From an early age, I worried about my sleep. I made an effort to be in bed on time. I had this internal clock that just said, "Time for bed!" As an adult, I am still similar to the young girl that is all grown up. Little did I know this would play an important part in my health, mood and schedule for each day.

Our sleeping habits affect our moods and our energy. With lack of sleep, well, you might miss out on carving out an exciting future if you are too tired to live life properly. The older I become, the more I have realized that following the correct rhythm of time is extremely important for how your feelings and your relationships play out on a day-to-day basis. You might be wondering how sleep ended up in the 'Love' section and not under 'Live.' The answer is simple.

Love yourself enough to make rest and sleep part of your schedule.

Love yourself and your loved ones enough to plan time for your sleeping patterns so you are not acting like a beastly animal because you are only operating on a few hours of sleep. Undo your sporadic sleep habits and unlock a new sense of happiness.

How Lack of Sleep Affects Your Health

According to a study done at Harvard: "Scientists have gone to great lengths to fully understand sleep's benefits. In studies of humans and other animals, they have discovered that sleep plays a critical role in immune function, metabolism, memory, learning, and other vital functions. The features in this section explore these discoveries and describe specific ways in which we all benefit from sleep." And also stating, "In the short term, a lack of adequate sleep can affect judgment, mood, ability to learn and retain information, and may increase the risk of serious accidents and injury. In the long term, chronic sleep deprivation may lead to a host of health problems including obesity, diabetes, cardio-vascular disease, and even early mortality."

This is a pretty obvious one, really, but I feel it's important to mention. Especially now in a world of technology, of smart-phones, tablets, and video games. Did you know that all of these gadgets reduce our brain's melatonin productivity, which is essential for good rest? These lights may seem like nothing to you, but you must remember also that leaving these lights on "cues the brain to stay awake in the evening."

So do yourself a favor and set new rules in the house, even for yourself:

Put your tablets and smartphones and computers and televisions away at least an hour before bed. Make quiet time for yourself instead. Be with your loved ones or take time to do some quiet deep breaths or meditating to help quiet your mind.

Sleep sounds rather boring. It seems to be a bother at times, too. But honestly, it's what we need in order to function properly and live a happier and upright life.

So don't slack on the sleep. Love yourself enough to get proper rest. Turn off the gadgets and get to bed. This is a gentle reminder to love yourself more by giving yourself more rest.

And yes, I am guilty of burning the candles at both ends on occasion. I have been one of those late-night owls who like to stay up late in the wee hours of the morning. I think there may be a correlation with our childhood in how we still feel as adults as if we are 'getting away with something.' What I do is allow myself one night a week to stay up late (if I know I can sleep in). I can hear you naysayers out there: "What a bore! Sleep? Ugh." If you are thinking this as you are reading, please just know you can turn your thoughts around and learn to love a routine that takes better care of the most important person in your world. YOU. Remember the wise words of the Dalai Lama. So what are you going to do tonight? *Get some extra shut-eye.* Life is too short to be grumpy because you are walking around sleep-deprived.

Solitude

This was my moment to look for the kind of healing and peace that can only come from solitude.
~ Elizabeth Gilbert

I can reflect back to my early days of walking around the streets of San Francisco and learning one of my greatest lessons in life: Solitude is good for the soul. I found out the hard way, like most of us do. I managed to leave my quaint small town back in Missouri and follow my heart to the bigger cities that lit the way of my dreams. I will never forget how alone I felt and the quiet space that frightened the younger me. I had always been in the family comfort of those who loved me. When I wasn't busy doing my auditions or my modeling bookings, sometimes I would browse around in the comfort of a grocery store. I would take my time staring at the different canned goods. I would read the back ingredients. And I remember feeling oddly strange because I found comfort there under the bright lights in the aisles of the grocery store. I would then buy one thing. I specifically remember buying this green pesto pasta in a plastic container and standing at the bus stop eating it alone. The concrete sidewalks, paved streets and hills could not quiet the restless loneliness I felt deep in my soul. But through these first six months on my own, I learned to be brave. I learned to endure the quiet. I learned that within the silence of solitude I became my own best friend.

Now, 23 years later, I can look back over my life and I can actually find that the memories of solitude and alone time have been peak moments of a shift—a new beginning of something bigger to come.

So now it seems as if it is so much more challenging to find space and quiet time in our lives. With so much technology and social media, who ever really feels lonely? But too much of that can be a false sense of belonging. So it's more important than ever that we make a space and take time for solitude. You must make peace with the quiet and learn to love. Solitude can become your best friend and show you how to be brave and teach you life lessons you never knew you were capable of handling.

According to psychologist Sherrie Bourg, "Solitude can enhance your quality of relationships with others." She also states,

By spending time with yourself and gaining a better understanding of who you are and what you desire in life, you're more likely to make better choices about who you want to be around. You also may come to appreciate your relationships more after you've spent some time alone.

Start incorporating more space for time to be quiet and alone. Learn how to embrace the pause of life—the slow period—and learn to make time to unfold the balance of what you want and what you need. Find out what your dreams are and discover certain aspects of your personality you may have been neglecting.

Albert Einstein also had his two cents on why solitude is essential to our souls: "The monotony and *solitude* of a quiet life stimulates the creative mind."

So get busy and find some time for solitude and embrace the quietness of your soul. Love yourself enough to allow this gift, even if it's just a walk in the park, to quiet your mind and find a moment...alone.

Sacrifice

Once there was a tree, and she loved a little boy.
~ Shel Silverstein, *The Giving Tree*

Just sharing that quote brought tiny tears to the corner of my eyes. This beloved classic children's book is in essence a fable to set us off on the right course in life and remember to give great sacrifice in order to find happiness and love.

Make sure you are giving parts of yourself to others. You know what I mean by that? Be real. Show something from the inside. Don't just put on the poker face and be a person that is merely going through the motions. Give more of yourself. Don't just always want things to go your way. Be willing to give up in an argument even if you think you could be or know you are right. Be willing to hand over the spotlight. Learn to be quiet. Learn to find ways to make others happy around you. This is in essence only making small sacrifices in your life compared to real sacrifice. *Sometimes the little battles are the biggest because we deal with them daily*. Listen more when someone is telling you a story. Don't be waiting for the end. Try to really hear what they are telling you. They are taking a moment to share their story, a little piece of their soul with you for the day. Do look up at the grocery store. Do smile. Say thank you. Don't always share your political opinions in the midst of opposition. Keep a smile and learn to care more for others' feelings and don't worry about 'trying to prove a point.'

The Merriam Webster Dictionary states:

sac·ri·fice: *The act of giving up something that you want to keep especially in order to get or do something else or to help someone*

Make time for the elders in your life. Take time to make them happy. Make time for those you love the most. Dare to give more of yourself on your journey. In turn, this will bring you more happiness. Also, don't impose your moods on everyone around you. Keep them to yourself. A mood is sure to pass. *A relationship is worth keeping.* So make sure you are caring more for your relationship with others than the right to project what you are feeling.

So What Are the Three S's?

- Sleep
- Solitude
- Sacrifice

At the end of the book *The Giving Tree*, the little boy is an old man and he sits on the stump. "And the tree was happy." *Life is meant to be shared, to be filled with love and compassion.* So have a heart and sacrifice a little of your own wants and needs to make someone else happy. The rewards are worth it.

We are all in the gutter, but some of us are looking at the stars.
~ Oscar Wilde

Chapter 20

One More Day Can Make the Difference. Keep Looking toward the Heavenly Stars

I am not sure why you picked up this book. Maybe you are searching for happier moments in your life. Maybe you are looking for an easy, quick fix to the pain you may feel deep down within your heart. I hope that some of my suggestions, interviews and stories can steer your heart into the light. My hope is that you can guide your own soul deep within to find your own guiding light.

Today, though, my heart is heavy. A beloved actor from my childhood memories has died from suicide. He was a brilliant actor. Yes, today is that day. And you may now be reading this looking back, remembering where you were when you heard the news that our favorite comedian died in the summer of 2014.

My question to you, dear reader: do you love those who surround you? Do you care enough to live one more day for them? If you are grappling with suicide or thinking it may be an easy way out, just remember all those who love you and will be forever left in your wake, your aftermath, your choice of turning out the lights when it was too soon for your death.

This journey is not easy. We slip. We fall. We falter and we even lose those we love. All that we know can crumble. We may have to rebuild from the foundation up. Our tragedies may have no rhyme or reason. There may be no answers for the pain you or I could be feeling in our hearts.

But think of this life. This beautiful moment of breath you were given to love, to think, to be, to have, to become anyone you want in this world. Think of all the incredible possibilities ahead of you.

Believe in them.

Believe in one more day.

Make it one more day. Have the courage to live one more day, not for yourself but for those who love you.

Be strong. Find that courage to be bold, dashing and charismatic. Think kinder words to your soul. Think brighter thoughts about your future.

This life is meant to be lived, explored, remembered, shared, to feel and to find what is really important.

I am so saddened by the death of my favorite actor that I loved so much. Yet I am more saddened for those who are left behind to make sense of what happened to him in the end.

My prayers are there for them.

So please have a heart. Have a kind, loving heart. Do think of those who may need you. Life, yes, can be cruel. But stay vigilant. Call on the angels. Believe in the hope that there is a brighter future for you—and guess what? It could even be tomorrow.

I remember after losing my friend to suicide, I was submerged in grief for some time. All our friends disbanded because of grief. My happy place became a place that marked memories of a time I could no longer access. I remember waking up to the sunny mornings wondering how life could still look so beautiful when the pain inside covered all in an eternal feeling of gray. Life went on, but my sunny heart had been saddened. I could not comprehend or understand why my friend left his world. I felt compassion for my friend and wished his soul well on crossing into Heaven. I do believe in that sort of thing. I do.

I did all of those things. But that pain was hard to bear.

If you are having issues in your life that could be suicidal, do reach out for help. Tell someone! Believe me, *they do care*. Don't hide your depression in a closet. Bring it out in the open. Ask someone to help you find a counselor, a pastor, a confidant who can help you recover your smile.

You can find it again. You must believe that your life, *your soul*, has a meaning and a purpose. You are here for a reason. Maybe you are meant to be that encouraging person to someone you have never met, yet. You heart will be that healer for someone else in time. You must know that you are special. God loves you. You are brilliant. Seek help. In the back of this book is a list of suicide hotlines for you to call.

Be bold and make the right decision…not for your loved ones, but for your beautiful soul. You might have to struggle to fight for your right to be happy again. But you can and will feel the sunlight on your face, if you can just make it one more day. One more to discover a new blessing and the answer to your pain.

All hope is not lost.

The darkness is only temporary. You will find your smile again. Love yourself. Be your own best friend.

Here are three quotes that explain in a deeper value the reason we may feel pain and why we must continue anyway.

You Are a Treasure

A pearl is a beautiful thing that is produced by an injured life. It is the tear that results from the injury of the oyster. The treasure of our being in this world is also produced by an injured life. If we had not been wounded, if we had not been injured, then we will not produce the pearl.
~ Stephan Hoeller

Development of Character

Character cannot be developed in ease and quiet. Only through experience of trial and suffering can the soul be strengthened, ambition inspired, and success achieved.
~ Helen Keller

147

Take Action

Action may not always bring happiness; but there is no happiness without action.
~ Benjamin Disraeli

I am just like you. I am human. I am fallible. I make mistakes. I must carry on through the hurt and the pain. I promise you, though, if you don't give up hope and if you believe in something new, you can develop a new future. You will breathe a sigh of relief. You will feel the light step under your feet. Your world will come together again and make sense. When we fall apart, something new and marvelous can spring forth and grow. A beautiful new development of hope can give us a deeper understanding of who we are and why we are here. So don't give in to the darkness. Please push on! Please believe in one more day. *You are BEAUTIFUL.*

Some people are settling down, some people are settling, and some people refuse to settle for anything less than butterflies.
~ Candace Bushnell, Author of *Sex and the City*

Chapter 21

Interview—with Matchmaker Elle France on Why Matters of the Heart...Matter

What does your love life look like? Are you in a rough patch, feeling blue or disheartened? Or are you one of those jaded types who stereotype men, or a man who stereotypes a woman into a certain category? Whether we like it or not, choosing our mate— when it comes down to it—is the most important decision that we make in terms of happiness. You don't have to be in a relationship to 'be happy.' Some think that happiness only exists behind a white picket fence or after the big fat white dress is displayed at the pulpit and then there is a cake to cut later. Some might think that spooning someone as they cuddle in bed is the only type of real love to chase after.

However, with that being said, some of the happiest and fun moments I have ever had were when I was single. So what we must remember before we forge ahead into a relationship is to make sure it's one where we will flourish, find peace, and enjoy this life with the other person as a teammate. This person should add a sense of comfort and safety, while embracing your wishes and dreams. I felt in this case, since matchmakers seem to be a staple in US society and their actual business is *'matters of the heart,'* why not go to the source for the inside scoop on dating, love and why it's a BIG ONE that matters?

Matchmaker Elle France has gained worldwide press for co-founding the SingldOut.com website that combines DNA and professionals who have LinkedIn profiles. Her 'Jerry Maguire' approach to matchmaking in Southern California has made her a sought-after interviewee in the matters of love.

Here is my interview with Matchmaker, Elle France:

What advice would you give to those looking for love when they are searching for their 'soul mate'? Do you believe there is such a thing that can resemble that in our modern society?

Matchmaker, Elle France: Even with all the social media and online dating, you can still do the things you love in order to meet someone. I believe that you can't let that person get by you that might spark your interest, whether it's at a coffee shop or a grocery store. There is too much temptation out there right at a person's fingertips with their phone, so if you want to find someone who is based on that instant chemistry, then you need to act on it. No bio on an online dating site or browsing through someone's Facebook photos can replace the chemical attraction when you meet someone who 'turns you on.' It doesn't mean that it is going to turn into a romantic relationship but it does mean that there is that natural human-to-human response that we are supposed to feel for someone who we want to get to know better. Technology has definitely changed the way we meet and date.

What do you find is the biggest mistake that tends to be repeated by many on their first date?

Matchmaker, Elle France: I know everyone is given rules on a first date. Don't drink too much. Don't talk about your ex. Don't call or text and don't talk about yourself all night long. If a person does any or all of these things, I would much rather know now than wait until the third date, or two months in, that they were putting on an act. The phony behavior can waste a lot of time. I would say, bait someone to find out who they are rather than having them put on an act. I realize people get nervous/excited when they first meet. There is a natural tendency to hold back a little or say things maybe that shouldn't be said on a first date. I am not so sure there is a mistake if people could just act how they really are feeling on the inside with a new person. My advice is: have fun, relax and take an interest in someone as you would want them to take an interest in you.

Why do you think love can be elusive for so many? Are they looking in the wrong places? What advice could you give on believing in first loves and second chances?

Matchmaker, Elle France: There are too many choices out there so it is overwhelming to the brain, especially with online dating. The pool of people who are available to you at one time is not normal. People tend to not take time with one person now, because of all the choices. They just think "Next!" and keep looking. And they are right. There is a 'next' right at their fingertips. But in the process of going to the next option, they may be missing out on someone wonderful right in front of them. So take time and get to know someone before you become fickle and want to move on.

Do you think that individuals can find love at any age, even after bad break-ups?

Matchmaker, Elle France: For first loves and second chances. It all depends on what broke them up in the first place, and how long they have been apart before trying again. If they have been apart for a while, it would be tough to put things back. Especially if you have dated in between. This always seems to haunt you. If you are honestly just taking a break to think and not get new people involved, then there is a chance, possibly. People tend to stay together for the wrong reasons if they keep breaking up. Most people don't want to go through the whole process again or don't want to be alone. But they still aren't happy staying together. You have to be uncomfortable in life at times in order to get out of a bad or unhappy situation. This is the only way to move forward.

What advice can you give someone who is starting over after their heart feels like it has been broken?

Matchmaker, Elle France: This is one thing that pretty much all humans have in common. You need to mourn for a reasonable time and then you need to start to occupy your mind with things that make you feel good. There is no way to not feel sad or bad at some point. Working out, exercising of any kind, will help release the hormones that make you feel good. I believe that you can find love over and over again. There is someone out there for everyone. That's what is so great about life. We do have choices. And no matter what choice you make, even if it's a wrong choice, you will have a chance to begin again.

Do you feel that having a personal relationship with yourself adds to someone's chances of connecting with a new love? And how do you feel about opposites? Should you try to find someone more like you? Or is that old adage, 'Opposites attract,' more accurate?

Matchmaker, Elle France: I definitely feel that you need to be in the right state of mind for things to go your way more. But I also believe that we all have stresses that happen to us and we can't predict when they will happen. You can find love or just someone you like at any point, even if you are at a tough point. They might be there for that purpose to help you out of a hard time in your life. I do not believe opposites attract for a long-term relationship. You need to stay with a like-minded person in order to keep you stimulated. For instance, if I am 'very hyperactive and very fast-paced,' I don't need someone to calm me down—I need someone to keep up. If he wants to get on the freeway and keeps getting in the slow lane and I want to move to the fast, I am going to feel like having a panic attack stuck in the slow lane. It's not going to work in the end. It will not be stimulating for you. This is not to say that what I feel as the opposite isn't true. Many couples are different and make their relationship work. I just think the first equation tends to work the best.

Any last thoughts that might help someone build their confidence when it comes to finding love, and what little rituals in your life do you do to make yourself happy?

Matchmaker, Elle France: I think we all deserve and want that feeling that we get when meeting someone. But sometimes that initial feeling changes. Don't let outside influences make you feel that you need something better. Misery loves company. There is no way that you are going to feel bliss 100% of the time. The times that you don't feel it, don't make the mistake of getting it from someone else. If you really love someone, and you know what that is, then cherish and protect it. I like to make sure that when I do go on walks, when I do walk through this life, that I take it all in and realize how very lucky I am to be here. I love *love*! I love that we have control over what we say and do, which can make all the difference in bettering our relationships. I also realize that I have no power to change someone or make them conform to me. My favorite ritual is looking in my dog's eyes and truly realizing the love that another life can give you unconditionally. Oh, if we could all be as happy and sweet as a dog!

I hope that insightful interview with Elle has given you an example of how you need to 'raise the bar' when it comes to love matters. So do be selective. Don't be fickle. Make sure you are giving someone who might really like you a fair chance. Don't always be looking for what is next. Make sure you don't miss the love of your life because you are too busy looking and not seeing what could be right in front of you.

Be present in your relationships. Cultivate them. Cherish them. And be your beautiful self.

Say your prayers and believe in attracting that certain someone who will add to your journey. In the meantime, enjoy being single. Enjoy your girlfriends or guy friends. Get busy living and exuding your inner light. While you weren't looking, someone might be watching, someone who might just become The One.

So don't fret. Be single. And enjoy your relationship with yourself. Life is not always about being with another person. It's also about learning to love the inner you and the journey of discovering hidden treasures buried deep inside. So make sure you are not just always *out there* looking. Have fun and love who you are along the way. You never know, that someone special might be in your next chapter. Just make sure you are enjoying this moment of being single, too.

Empathy is really the opposite of spiritual meanness. It's the capacity to understand that every war is both won and lost. And that someone else's pain is as meaningful as your own.

~ Barbara Kingsolver

Chapter 22

Empathy and Why We Need More of It

The clouds are dangling low over the Denver airport. I am in between planes and in between thoughts. Life is a delicate balance. With the recent losses of Malaysian Airlines Flight 370 (still missing in late 2014) and the ferry that sank in South Korea, which claimed the lives of almost 300 students in one high school, my heart is heavy with grief. My heart breaks for those in the Midwest and the South of the USA who just lost everything in violent tornadoes. This list does not end.

This life is a mystery. We just truly do not know what tomorrow brings.

I want to reach out here as I sit in the Denver airport and write this chapter. I want to pause and send my prayers and condolences to all those beautiful families in South Korea, to the parents of soldiers who never came home, to those who have lost loved ones due to a sudden accident or disease. I wish I could do something to make your pain for your loved one subside. I wish you love and light, and that your grief will abate with the passing years.

As I was sitting here, I came across another story of a mother who just lost her two young sons in the recent tornadoes. She sent out a message of light and faith for those to hear. She is relying on God and Christ and putting her grief in Their Hands. She shared a picture of herself in her hospital bed with her face cut up, battered and bruised. She bravely held a photo of the family she just lost in the storm. She wanted to share on social media her bravery and love for those she had just lost. Her courage must be commended and recognized. I salute her strength and her faith in God.

Life Must Go On

This journey is not always fair. Tragedies happen every day. So we must learn to have more empathy for others and their plight. Have more empathy for those who have lost. Choose to feel for them, carry a moment of their sorrow. Feel their pain. Be human enough to care and not the type of human to turn your back the other way. It is important that we honor and respect our fellow loved ones walking this earth. Everyone has their own cross to bear. And sometimes we must bear their pain, too. Show that we care and that we understand. And it's good to grieve for those who need it. Do not turn your back on the sorrows of this world. Be human enough to care and to give part of your soul. *What is your reward?* By sending loving thoughts and prayers, you have paused to give part of you to their struggle. You have taken a brief moment to send loving energy to someone who needs it. You paused from your blessings to remember someone else's sorrows, which will remind you of how this life is such a precious gift...each day!

Do not numb yourself to pain. Instead, open the floodgates. Have the courage to give something of yourself to make this world a better place.

Be a person who cares! Life can be short. Dare to feel someone else's pain.

Experience the beauty of emotion. Do not close yourself off to what Mother Teresa taught us best. She was just one woman who exemplified the power of empathy by removing herself from the equation. Her compassion and vulnerabilities touched the sick and those whom the rest of society would deem unworthy. Mother Teresa looked inside and saw the beating of the human heart. We can do the same, too. This world is in need of our caring, our sharing and our empathy. So don't numb yourself to pain or the pain of others. Be open to carry their grief and share in the hard experiences, too. Open your soul to feeling more than just what you want to feel. When we open ourselves to caring for others, our return benefit is just this:

We become part of the human experience and not just a selfish person after our own selfish wants and needs.

On our quest for happiness, let us not forget to shoulder the burden of our friends in need, our neighbors who might need us, or our loved ones. Even reach out to a stranger who may look distraught. Offer a smile, a warm heart. See if there is something you can do to unload a tiny bit of their burden. Life is not just about traipsing down the lane of bliss. Lend your heart and your hand when you can. Open up to the beautiful possibility that you have the power to help another, and do so. In the loving words of Mother Teresa, "I have found the paradox, that if you love until it hurts, there can be no more hurt, only more love."

What can you do to develop more empathy?

- Listen more to others.
- Be more caring and attentive to your inner circle.
- Practice praying for others always, even for strangers you might have met on the street.
- Write down in your journal why empathy can improve your relationships.
- Practice self-love, which will in turn give you more love to give.
- Read. Learn from great teachers.
- Go visit a homeless shelter. Experience other walks of life that can shine a light on the human experience we are all living.
- Write down in your journal all that you are grateful for and list those whom you love. Say a prayer for them and

imagine their world in a painless place.

I must remind myself of these things to do, too. I must work on keeping myself connected to the human experience, and show and feel compassion. I hope that you can open your heart, and send love, even if just for a small, short moment. This world is in need of more compassion and love.

Part Three—Soul

Believe in yourself and all that you are. Know that there is something inside you that is greater than any obstacle.
~ Christian D. Larson

Why should we think upon things that are lovely? Because thinking determines life. It is a common habit to blame life upon the environment. Environment modifies life but does not govern life. The soul is stronger than its surroundings.
~ William James

Be careless in your dress if you must, but keep a tidy soul.
~ MarkTwain

Happiness resides not in possessions, and not in gold; happiness dwells in the soul.

~ Democritus

Chapter 23

Have a Little *Soul*

You could say I am sort of obsessed with the soul. Our soul. Your soul. Our souls call out to us in the dark of the night with our deepest fears and with our brightest light. Our soul knows right from wrong. Our soul remembers the simple vignettes of the waves washing over our feet on the sand. It lingers in the memories, wishing for more love, more nourishment, more thought and...what? *More soul.*

In a world that is leading us into a phone-obsessed culture or the next best gadget, we must make sure to remember who we are, what we love, and open our hearts to our friends and family. We must remember to share our soul.

I found out a lot about soul work, believe it or not, as a reader and an actress. I followed the path of uncovering what made characters work and why they felt emotions. I wanted to dig in and get to the bottom of the 'why' in life. I searched in my twenties for something more meaningful. I needed to root out the monkey chatter of my smaller thoughts and believe there was something higher calling me to a purpose in life.

What does it all mean really, this life? To be good, to be kind, to be loving and to show compassion. Feel something. Add something to this life. Don't just be one those individuals who are sitting on the sidelines.

In this section, I am going to share with you some of my own trials and tribulations and little methods and exercises that have helped me find more inner peace and happiness.

I added three quotes at the beginning of the 'Soul' section because this section is what the book is ultimately about: YOU. The innermost desires of your heart and what you are trying to be in this world. In order to find your peace and joy within your own space, you must first know who you are. What do you love? What are your ambitions? What are your secret, private joys? How can you attain that one dream that just might seem out of reach?

In the 'Soul' section:

- Crafting the story of your life and your book cover
- An interview with a Zen teacher on the 'power of your core'
- An interview with Soul Icon and violinist, Lindsey Stirling
- Why taking care of your home and personal things adds joy to your daily routine
- Why exercise and diet are essential to your soul
- Making time for Mother Nature
- An interview with Dr Doris Lee McCoy
- A Soul Kit and a Safety Net—why you need both

I am excited that you are here with me. I hope you apply some of these exercises to help you find more love and happiness in your daily life. There is no shortage of joy in this world. We must uncover it first within ourselves. So many times we look for others and circumstances to make us happy. Our attachment to joy and dreams must first be planted deep within the center of our soul. We must find sturdy ground so that the changes and unforeseen circumstances we may not expect only sway us ever so slightly. This life is a gift. A moment. A dream. A story that we share with each other. My hope is to inspire you to find your light and how to defeat whatever threatens to rob you of your right to be happy. Our right to be happy is ours. We must just cultivate it, believe in it and want it. Why choose something else if we can outline and fill our hearts with a plan and a guide that can stabilize and keep our hearts merry?

So a few more questions before we move ahead:
1. When is the last time you sat down for teatime alone and examined your wants and needs?
2. Are you making quiet moments for yourself?
3. Are you taking time to reach within and connect with your inner voice, that deep intuition that can be an internal compass for your life?

These three questions may sound far-fetched and removed from the hectic-pace world we live in today. From our smartphones and tablets, to receiving our notification alert numerous times in the day, are you remembering to stay plugged into...you?

A little soul-searching can go a long way.

Let the gentle, wise words of Thomas Moore, the author of *Care of the Soul*, remind you of what's most important: "A genuine odyssey is not about piling up experiences. It is a deeply felt, risky, unpredictable tour of the soul." So remember to schedule a date with your soul. Remember to set some time aside and learn what really makes you tick from the inside out. If you don't have a clue how to do that, or are unsure of how to connect with your intuitive side, this book is for you. With little steps, easy actions and inspiring daily activities you will be stepping into your own dynamic soulful self, leading you to find the secrets to happiness by taking that exciting journey within. Just remember to leave your smartphone on the bedside table. It's time to get busy and find out some important factors that can and will brighten your day because you are making a decision to place *your soul* first. This takes love and heart. But I assure you, making time for a more meaningful and fulfilled life will help keep the boredom away and the fear of uncertainty. Be certain by knowing who and what you are. The rest will fall into place.

There is no greater agony than bearing an untold story inside you.
~ Maya Angelou

Chapter 24

The Power of Sharing and Honoring Each Other's Stories

It's too hot to write. I am sitting in the kitchen in Pauma Valley, California with an iced coffee inside a white mug. Next to the mug is a water spritzer with lavender oils. This is my one escape for beating the heat. I have been luxuriating in the quietness of the hills and this valley. Peacocks run wild here. I am on their soil. Their ground. They view me from outside of the little ranchhouse my husband's family owns. They watch my every move. Their brilliant peacock feathers of blues and greens and gray lie strewn across the land as souvenirs for the tourists. That would be me. I finally got a mini-getaway. This isn't Mexico. But it might as well be, with the dry heat and balmy air dancing through the citrus trees.

Earlier today, I took my Doberman for a walk underneath the hot sun as we scanned the orange groves for peacock feathers. We walked onto the base of the property where a little graveyard stands alone under two solid eucalyptus trees. Flags decorated the cemetery. Those lying there underneath the ground are part of the Pala tribe and maybe the Pauma tribe, too. This is their sacred land. We are here now, too. I walked along the edges of the cemetery, reading the headstones. I read them and felt their lives pass within my mind for a flickering second, revealing their story to me. Their story. What their lives were about. Where they slept, ate their food and shared their soul with those who might have loved them...or maybe they were not loved? What was their story?

Each story has a purpose to one generation. A lineage. A meaning. Those who sit next to us on an airplane or pass us on a crowded street in a downtown city carry their stories, too.

With much reflection for writing this book, I keep seeing the value of a story and why it is important to listen to others when they take time to share a piece of their lives with us. Maybe it's a moment. You might be at a check-out counter in a grocery store. You are in a hurry. You don't want to hear any words. Your day has just been one of those long drawn-out days that feel like too much, and you definitely don't have time for a stranger.

Well, perk up your ears. Lend a listen. Don't turn yourself away from their need to share what's on their mind with you. It could be a sliver of their life laid out with crayons tracing their origin. It might be that they had a bad day, too, and they want to commiserate with someone close to them, and it happens to be you.

Don't turn away from their story. Don't turn your soul silent to their needs. If you can, listen. Take an interest. This is their life they are touching upon yours with their words and their thoughts. It's a moment you may never have again. You may never see this person again. This moment is just a few minutes in time where two unknown souls meet. There is an opportunity for sharing, for caring and for taking time to honor someone's story.

I just felt a gentle breeze inside the yellow kitchen where I am sitting. The floor below me is hardwood. The air is melting the tiny beads of sweat on my back. This moment is my moment of sharing a sliver of my life with you. I married a wonderful man with a family that has a beautiful citrus ranch beneath the Palomar Mountains in California. The world is so quiet right now. I can see oranges dangling from the trees outside the window above the sink. My beloved Dobie is right next to my feet, curled up on a rug I laid out for him. He is rather warm today. This beauty might be too warm for us in Pauma Valley.

A peacock just cooed and there is always an eerie silence after they stop. I feel as if I am intruding on their privacy. Their camp. Their nest. They watch us with a steady head and sharp vision from afar. They wait for us to leave. I love their wild, beautiful bodies. The delicate, uncolored females without the glory the male wears. I love the sound of a rooster crowing from the backyard behind me. A neighbor nearby has roosters and hens for his family. Earlier this morning, when the sun was beginning to rise over the sleepy valley, I let my Dobie outside. He managed to leap away from the leash I was holding and chased the roosters and chickens. I watched them scatter underneath the citrus trees.

"Fortune," I cried out. "Fortune!! Stop!"

At the end of the driveway of the other home was the owner of the chickens and roosters. We shared a moment of our little worlds colliding. My dog had invaded his story. I felt a connection for a brief moment as he waved to me, like a signal not to worry.

Finally Fortune came back. I am here now. That was just a sliver of my day. Besides lying out on a wicker brown beach placemat under the hot sun for one hour, with my water bottle and my book. The sun melted away every single thought. There was nothing but heat on my back and pouring from my face. The power of the sun felt so exhilarating. Life was still around me except for the peacock calling.

Later I took a delicious cold shower. So cold, my body felt as if it had been revived for a moment from the heat.

In the middle of the day, I had to shut all the blinds, close the doors and make the ranch-house cooler with the pull-down shades.

Now I am back to you, dear reader. What is your story? Is it a good one? Do you like how it is going? Or are you unsatisfied with a few details that you wish you could change?

Take time right here in this empty space in the book to spell out, "If you had the power to change your story, what would it look like and how would you do it?"

What do you want to change?

Can you visualize what you wish you could make your life? If so, write it here.

Do you build castles to the sky with dreams that you wish to dream? If not, do so now here in this empty space. Connect your dream with your pen or pencil and write it down. Make it tangible. Share your cherished wishes with your soul. Do so now.

What Is Your Story?

Do you know? An essential part of learning to grow and loving ourselves more is creating the story of the life we wish to live. This is your moment in the sun. This is your moment to create *anything*. Take time to make your life what you want it to be. Write down your story and get to know yourself. There is nothing more important than the power of a story. From mythology, to history set before us, or by uncovering fossils hidden beneath the sand, each living thing has a story of its own.

You do, too. Make sure you are the creator and not just a visitor in your own land. Don't just watch your life unravel like a loose yarn or thread out of control. You control it.

Before I finish up this chapter, I must share with you what inspired me to add this chapter to *Live Love Soul* and why it's an important *piece of peace* in your life. I, as I have been writing this book, have been watching others and listening more. I want to find out their slices of joy and if they are happy or sad. I find people fascinating from all walks of life. (Must be the old actress girl in me that loves a good story.)

Well, about two months ago, I met an elegant woman at my husband's gift and produce shop in Rancho Santa Fe. She started telling me about how she liked to make organic chocolates. Each weekend she would reveal something new to me. Eventually, I began sharing pieces of my story with her, too. I gave her my book, *Middle Age Beauty*, as a gift. She took time to read it. Then the following weekend, I found out she was a neurophysicist and professor at Caltech University in Pasadena. Imagine! Next she brought by a sample of a new book she was writing. I took it out of the yellow manila envelope and handled it with care. How special of her to share these pages of her life with me! It was her memoir, filled with beautiful pictures of her life, too.

I haven't seen her in a while. I am eagerly waiting to tell her how her story of a young girl coming to school in America from Europe touched me with hope and innocence. I want to tell her I loved her love story of how she met and fell in love with her husband. And how they stayed married until the end of his life, had two daughters, and rode horseback together holding hands in an open field somewhere in California.

I want to tell her that her story reached inside my soul and found pieces of myself in it. I found a piece of my heart beating the same as hers, with the same wants and desires.

Having compassion and honoring our own story, while embracing others with theirs with an open heart...well, this might be one of the most important things you do in your life. To learn to reach out, step outside of your comfort zone and tune into the stories around you. You might just discover an untapped piece of your soul you never recognized before. Sometimes it takes another person to mirror our own life and reveal what we cannot see without their help.

Now the air is still in the kitchen here in the valley. The peacocks are silent. I am nostalgic for my friend that I have not seen in a while. I want to hug her and say thank you for sharing her life with me. It opened up a new part of myself with a happiness I have not known.

This life can be terribly short. So make sure you are tuning into the stories that fill your life. Make sure you are the creator of your own. Life can fall away from us just like a cemetery can remind us of the passage of time. Life can be fleeting. Our time on earth is precious. So use it wisely. Love and create a story that you will be proud to leave behind. Also, make time to honor the stories of those you love and those you do not know. You might be surprised at what you find when you just take time to hear a new story that you do not know. So get busy and start listening.

Whenever I feel blue, I start breathing again.
~ Frank L. Baum, Author of *The Wonderful Wizard of Oz*

Chapter 25

Interview—with Author and Zen Life Coach, Michiko Jane Rolek

As I laid out in the last chapter, sharing our stories helps us to feel more compassion and learn more about ourselves, and this is exactly what happened to me when I met my mentor and life coach Michiko Jane Rolek. Michiko was referred to me by a friend during my early twenties. I was living in Studio City, at the time a working commercial actress and model. I had been living in Los Angeles for about six years, I think, when I hit upon a deep void on my journey. My footing felt off and I was smart enough to seek guidance. Little did I know that the person I was about to meet would change my life with her exquisite grace, language of love, and the power of deep breathing. If you want, throw in the word 'meditation.' Yes, that's what it was, but more accessible than hours on a floor. She taught me mini-breathing exercises that I could apply to my daily routine. I found immediate release from the fear and stress I was experiencing. Michiko also helped me to discover the 'power of my core' and why it's essential to stay connected to it when it comes to meditating, and standing with posture. Working with her as a life coach helped me shift my fear and insecurities into action and strength. And it all began with learning the value of my core (the area where your stomach and just below your ribcage meet on your body).

Here is my interview with Michiko today. I am still blessed with her shining light, her guiding hand, and her spirit like a sparkling diamond that has been so influential. Thank you, Michiko, for your love. And here in her own words, you will understand more of the meaning of 'the core—your core' and why you need to learn more about it on your journey to happier moments.

Please explain why the core of our bodies is such an important part of our body and our spiritual center. You refer to this as our 'diamond core.' Why?

Michiko J. Rolek: The diamond *core* is associated with Zen training. Most precious things lose their value or meaning if they're broken, but if a diamond is cut into smaller pieces, each facet is still valuable.

With core strengthening, we keep this in mind: a little bit of practice goes a long way to help us shift from a worrier to a warrior, wearing our black belt for the soul. By directing the stream of our breath to our diamond core, we dissolve stress, worries, anger, and tension, transforming negativity into clear positivity. Like spiritual alchemy, a diamond is coal transformed, so calm clarity can arise from chaos and confusion. The *core* is located at the center of the body, measuring from top to toe. That still point is located about 2–3 inches below the navel. Our entire body is coordinated from this center of balance, physically, mentally, and emotionally.

What can someone do to become more aware of the core in their normal activities every day? Why do you think it's more common for many (including myself) to want to slouch forward instead of holding our shoulders back in alignment with our spine and core center?

Getting in touch with our core in everyday activities starts with becoming aware of our posture and breathing habits throughout the day. Keep in mind that proper posture encourages proper breathing. Our body's 'core' or center-line is just as it is for an apple. These deep core muscles include our abdomen, back and pelvis; they provide our structural base of stability, like a deeply rooted tree. The good news is that by strengthening our core, the rest of the body follows. The reason many people slouch is because their body-soul instrument hasn't been trained to straighten up and fly right. My first book, *Mental Fitness*, offers useful tools to master the fundamentals, using fun as creative fuel to turn obstacles into learning opportunities.

Here's my favorite posture pointer to practice during your activities of daily living: walking, sitting at a computer, standing in line, driving: Think of your spine as the stem and your head as a blossoming flower. Become mindfully aware of the tail end of your spine and your chin. If either one is sticking out excessively, it is like the root or the rose being cut off from the stem.

Now, sink your roots and blossom where you land, one breath at a time...ahhhh.

You have mentioned to me in our previous classes together that 'society as a whole' are shallow breathers. Most are unaware of their breathing and if they are even breathing properly. What simple exercise can you give as an example here that could help someone develop better breathing skills?

Michiko J. Rolek: Simply observing your breath non-judgmentally is the first step towards practicing mindful breath awareness, which creates the right conditions for the breathing process to become less shallow and more steady on its own. Our spiritual muscle is the diaphragm; consider how the word 'spirit' means 'to breathe.' The In-breath is inspiration; the Out-breath, expiration. When we are breathing correctly, which I clarify in *Mental Fitness*, which has been fondly called 'Yoga off the Mat', like ocean waves, the tummy (abdomen) rises on the inhalation and falls on the exhalation.

Remember, when your breathing is relaxed and rhythmic, your mind naturally becomes calm and clear. The word *Hara* (located in the lower abdomen) in Japanese means 'ocean of energy or light.'

Can you explain the importance of our breath and how it can affect our health, mood and ability to think clearly?

Michiko J. Rolek: I often refer to breathing as our magic mood-booster. When we are breathing high in our chest or taking shallow breaths, our stress level increases, and the energy is low, leaving us feeling helpless and exhausted. We can correct this immediately by breathing with our diaphragm, our spiritual muscle. In up to 3–6 breaths we can interrupt the stress pattern of anxiety and depression. Here's how: As the diaphragm moves, it relaxes upwards expelling stale air on the Out-breath, and contracts downwards expanding the lung capacity on the In-breath. On the Out-breath the abdomen contracts, flattens towards the spine; as the diaphragm relaxes and rises on the exhalation, it sends an 'All is well' message to the brain. What follows is a brighter mood, with the potentiality to think clearly with less anxiety and more serenity.

What other advice can you give for simple exercises on developing 'core' strength and 'core' awareness? Do you think there is a link to a better sense of well-being?

Michiko J. Rolek: Yes, there is a connection to our happiness, initiated from mindful awareness and exercising to build core strength. When we feel positive about our bodies growing stronger, focused on our purpose, we can get along better with others, which in turn enhances our well-being. The Zen approach that I successfully use every day is called The

Miracle Diamond of Mindfulness; it's a secret dancer's posture habit that helps us find balance in the dance of life. Being mindful is simply returning to our breath and posture in the present moment, non-judgmentally with compassionate attention.

Here's a soul recipe to polish your Miracle Diamond in three easy-as-pie steps.

1. Get Grounded: sink your roots by pressing your sit bones or feet down to feel centered in the here and now.
2. Be Grateful: spread your heart wings by softening your shoulders, keeping your head to the sky.
3. Hello Gorgeous: getting grounded and grateful awakens your authenticity so your soul can glow, and the true 'you' can shine through brilliantly.

You have taught many celebrities and received famous endorsements from world-renowned spiritual leaders and authors with your simple and realistic approach to meditation, which is steeped in legacy and ancestry. If someone has never meditated, why should they learn and how can they incorporate simple meditation exercises?

Michiko J. Rolek: Simply put, Zen means meditation; it helps us get in touch with our souls and connects us with our spirit. Working with famous stars is a lil' slice of heaven. Because in most cases they're ready to dig in, and respect the work in progress of keeping Zenergized calm, to do the hustle, and sparkle on, both personally and professionally. Everyone is born with the enlightened seed of joy and having a clear mind, peaceful heart. It is up to us to nurture our heart's garden.

To easily incorporate a little Zen into your activities of daily living, and water the soul seed of happiness already in you, here's a magical single-breath meditation that I practice with my daughter, Grace, every day. Let's Tune-out, Tune-in, and Tune-up with a One Breath, Zen Tune-up:

Tune-out: *Whoosh…exhale stale air and release any distraction — scattered mental energy.*

Tune-in: *Focus on your mindful breath which is your anchor to stay present, smile.*
(pixie pause to reach stillness)

Tune-up: *Let it go… Ahhh… See differently with your worrier to warrior spirit of a clear mind, peaceful heart. Carry this gem of Zen wisdom: focus on one thing at a time to stay present and clear-headed moment by moment. The miracle is, at any moment we can begin again.*

So get busy breathing. Learn and teach yourself to become a deep breather. Get that extra oxygen to your blood cells. Calm your mind. Silence that 'monkey chatter/spinning thoughts' that can get you down. Learn how to breathe again. Get connected to your breath. This is the best and most important tool I learned and developed to help alleviate my mind from fear. Thank you, Michiko Jane Rolek, for being my teacher and for sharing your inner words of wisdom and Zen lineage here within the pages of *Live Love Soul*. You are my earth angel.

Faith is to believe what you do not see; the reward of this faith is to see what you believe.
~ Saint Augustine

Chapter 26

Why Believing in Something Matters

The word 'soul' in itself can dredge up so much. Some think of it as an esoteric thing or New Age thing. But well-known author CS Lewis did not. One of his famous quotes, "You don't have a soul. You are a soul. You have a body," actually originated first from Scottish author George Macdonald who died in 1905. He said:

> *Never tell a child, you have a soul. Teach him, you are a soul. You have a body.*

Since we are on the topic of authors, I will share with you that I am an admirer of the woman who wrote the book featuring Julia Child. You know, the Julie/Julia writer who cooked 354 recipes from the ever-famous beloved Julia Child's French cookbook. I am thinking of her right now because when I reached the end of that fabulous memoir, the author shared that she didn't believe Julia Child was in Heaven. She clearly states that she is still in the casket buried under the dirt.

Okay.

Why give that image? Why take away the magnitude of how wonderful Julia Child was as a person, to keep her buried in the ground? She goes on to write that Julia does live on in memory. Isn't that the same?

No.

Quite frankly, it's not. I've never really understood the point of not having a belief system of some sort. I mean, don't you need some tools to help you through those darker moments? At some point we must all reach within and find something more than just ourselves. Because if that's it, I will admit it sounds a bit

185

depressing. Isn't that so?

So why you should expound a faith system:

I am well aware of the fact that I cannot prove to you that Christ or God exists. At least not here at this moment in this chapter. You are right. I have not been to Heaven. There might be the chance that when I die there is nothing but the dirt buried on top of my coffin. But so what? So what if that happens? In the meantime, I have faith, scripture and prayer to guide me through darker trials. I have a moral compass to guide me to work on having more compassion, and a light that adds comfort during dark days. What's so wrong with that?

I think nothing.

So for now, if you don't believe in God or Christ or the angels, just go with me here on this. Just open your mind to the possibility of the major *safety net* you are missing out on in your daily battles.

So, no offense to the author—I do think she is a wonderful writer. But I hated that version of our beloved Julia there. I would like to think of her with her soul mate, with Paul, in *Heaven*. So much more lovely, don't you think? And this is what I personally believe.

Life Can Be Tough

Right now, for example, I have had a hard month. Why? You know, I don't know why, but that's just been the brunt of it. Not hard like disease or tornadoes or hurricanes and such. But hard like in experiencing vertigo. I had suffered from a prolonged sinus infection that became an inner ear infection. The pain felt like my head was busting open from the seams. This caused the vertigo, which is a bout of dizziness. If I turned my head slightly, this pain filled my neck, my back and the sides of my temples. After a serious round of antibiotics, the vertigo had dissipated, but hadn't left my vision altogether. When I slept at night, my mind and dreams felt like a fun house with those mirrors and topsy-turvy floors.

I am sharing this with you because this is the first time in years I felt sheer utter fear that paralyzed my mind. I kept hearing this phrase, "The only thing to fear is fear itself."

What was my lesson? Show me the lesson! I so desperately wanted to be out of pain.

Yes, we all know that phrase about fear. *How do we conquer that big bad boy?*

GOD.

I turn to God. I pray. I reach in and reveal my most vulnerable self and offer up my weaknesses, my failures, my regrets, my wishes, and ask for help. I humble myself and ask for guidance and relief from fear and pain.

"Have mercy on my soul, Father. I trust you."

We all need a Father figure in this life. If you want to think of God as a woman, well, I know there are a few religions that embrace that theory. Whatever works for you. My point is that during this scary, unbalancing time, I found refuge in my faith. My prayers through meditations helped me alleviate much of my own inner fear, which was affecting my daily life. I had some tools and faith to take down the *big bad fear* to help me achieve a better day.

I don't like it when I am not on 'my game.' So when I am down, I truly dig deep within my soul to conquer the demons (figuratively speaking) that threaten to defeat me. You need to shed light on your own darkness in order to find a way out. We cannot be our only source of inspiration. Find God. Find a light. Find this beautiful place within yourself where you can connect and hear an inner voice guiding you when you need it the most.

These last few weeks have not been fun. When I was constantly walking around thinking I might have a brain tumor because the room was spinning, well, you could say I felt a bit distracted and uneasy. My book reading stopped. The only thing other than prayer that kept me grounded were my early morning nature hikes. There's nothing like getting out there and seeing the world up close and personal to enhance the positivity of your day. Even with life's physical aches and pains.

So back to the soul. Yes, your soul! You need to tend to it. You need to exercise it. You need to nourish the wants and needs that cry for your attention. If you walk around too long ignoring those cries, be prepared to have something soon level you to your knees…sort of like my bout with vertigo. (Yes, I saw that Grace Kelly movie.)

Many times we think we know our 'script.' We think we know the outcome of tomorrow. After all, won't it be just a repeat of next week and the next and the next?

No. We don't know that for sure. We only know that, God willing, the sun will rise again… Tomorrow is a mystery. Trust the mystery. Walk lighter on your feet. Find joy in knowing that what is here now may change to something even more lovely.

I will be honest with you. Yes, I can experience those humdrum times that lead me to a place that has my eyes finding the ground as I walk from task to task. My shoulders are heavy with burden. My day feels less than special and I wonder, "What's the point?" This is when we must take time to care for our soul and body.

If you don't want your world to be an emotional rollercoaster ride built on your 'emotion of the day,' you need to actively seek to find ways to connect deeper within and channel your desires and passions. You need to work on making your life more soulful. By your actions, by your planning. By your thoughts. Yes, you may still have a day when the world feels terribly bleak and you are unsure how you can take another step forward. You may wonder why you can't escape that crushing feeling that has stolen your joy.

I feel that when these times come, just as mine did with the bout of vertigo, there is a chance for much self-reflection and discovery. When we are not in sync and in tune with what is going on around us, we must be willing to make the journey within to find out why. I will admit that digging up the rocks in the rugged wilderness of the barren untapped parts of my soul is not that much fun. What is wonderful though, when these moments occur, is that I am able to connect with my faith in God. A higher being that is guiding me and making my journey a little less difficult.

So get ready to find ways to exercise, soothe and inspire your quiet self that needs some love. Get ready to find time, make time and enjoy making moments for just you. We all know that we must love ourselves. It's sort of cliché to even write that. (Yes, revisit that self-love chapter if you must for the lists of how self-love can empower your journey.) However, clichés can be built on repeated truths. There is a reason why we must find what delights our soulful existence. Soul work is not always easy. The hurt and the pain that we may have to face from years of ignoring wounds from yesterday are unpleasant to experience. But once we pull out the weeds and tend to our own garden, the effort of our works and attention to detail, which just happens to be *you*, will be so rewarding.

Thomas Moore, the author of *Care of the Soul* and many other books, states, "It may help us, in those times of trouble, to remember that love is not only about relationship; it is also an affair of the soul."

Back to Julia? I believe she is in Heaven living in a place that resembles Paris with her husband that she so loved. I believe they are there cooking up a storm and enjoying their reunion. Why not think happier thoughts?

Sometimes the others are too hard to bear. So get busy and find faith. Discover God and unload your daily burdens to give your day a bit more joy along the way. You might be surprised at what a little faith in something more than yourself can do for you...

If you don't know the trees, you may be lost in the forest; but if you don't know the stories, you may be lost in life.
~ Siberian Elder

Chapter 27

Designing the Book Cover of Your Life

When I was living in Hollywood in my early twenties I discovered a book that would soon go on to be one of the best 'self-publishing stories' in history, while impacting and changing lives. As a young 20-year-old finding her own way in the world, I had also found that I enjoyed reading 'self-help' books of all sorts. If you've ever been to Hollywood you could see how a town that breeds celebrity and blockbuster movies can breed insecurity in the most secure individuals. Usually with anyone that starts to fearlessly chase a dream there comes a point where you begin to hit roadblocks. Your initial thoughts of illusions behind what you were hoping for pale in comparison to what you were expecting. Welcome to reality, as they say. But because the contrast of your dream and the sharp real world can be two polar opposites, does that mean you should fling your dreams away? Does that mean you need to become more realistic and less dreamy?

I found myself at this set of crossroads when I was in my early twenties. The young dreamer girl had grown up and become a woman. I had followed my pursuit of modeling, which had been lucrative and exciting. I had moved from my small town in Southern Missouri to many cities all over the United States. Ultimately, though, after moving from city to city as a 'catalog' model, I decided to make Los Angeles my primary place of residence, which of course led to my agents leading me toward commercials and acting. Why not, I thought? After some easy success in booking an independent film, commercials and lucrative work, I soon fell prey to feeling insecure and wondering when this streak of good luck would end.

In search of understanding how I could flip from such confidence to sheer fear, I found myself inside one of the coolest bookstores in West Los Angeles, called The Bodhi Tree, a popular spiritual bookstore (this bookstore closed its doors after 40 years of business) and the mecca of the city. It was there that I found a book that predated the self-publishing business boom by almost 20 years: *The Celestine Prophecy* by James Redfield. This book went on to spend 165 weeks on the *New York Times* bestsellers list. These facts are only important to emphasize that it was not only myself that found some sort of comfort from this story. What was it about, in case you haven't read it? This book analyzed the power of energy and how we can adapt and pull the sources of energy from around us. It labeled four types of personalities that we all can primarily label ourselves and so gain knowledge from how we seek our own energy—an accumulative response, you might say—from those we interact with and apply it to the story we are building about our lives. When I applied these four personality archetypes to my personality, I found that I was petrified by the one I thought I fit under: 'Poor Me.' The Poor Me folks preyed on others' energy by making them feel guilty in order to gain attention.

I could blame this on being the third child in a line of siblings. I could blame this on the fact I lived alone and was unmarried and single in Hollywood. I was single in the city before Carrie Bradshaw became a household name. I found myself feeling vulnerable and exposed in a business that felt to me 'only skin deep.' Just like dreams and realities, what originally attracted me to being a model (travel and excitement) had now begun to wear down my steel backbone and expose weaknesses I had never known.

This period in my life became a restructuring of sorts. I found a manager. I left a huge acting agency for a smaller boutique agency. I gobbled up self-help books. I began reflecting on what my overall journey was about. I began to 'go within' in search of something more than just lipstick and my appearance. There had to be more to this world and I was going to find it.

Reading this book, *The Celestine Prophecy*, shifted my foundation. After discovering a flaw in my personality, I treaded toward rewriting my story. At that point, it had emulated 'a young model from the Midwest feeling vulnerable and alone in a big city.' Well, who wants to be that? Instead of building a pity fence around my realization, I took responsibility for my own actions and decided to rewrite my *headline*.

Life is a series of chapters that become our own personal book we write for ourselves.

You may not be picking up a pen or pencil and writing your life. But whether or not you are aware of it, your life right now is reflecting a story — Your Story. Sometimes life can happen in a set of circumstances that pushes you along swiftly without thought or action like a river flowing effortlessly. But when the drought comes and the riverbed dries up, you can find yourself stuck without knowing how you got there. When this happens and if this happens, the best thing to do before making a hasty decision is to reflect. Looking back, my hasty decision was to move to New York and change the scenery. This seemed like an exciting thing to do. But with deeper reflection I realized I would only be fleeing from a vulnerable feeling that would follow me to New York City.

I don't like feeling afraid, fearful or stuck. I don't think anyone does. In a world that prescribes a pill for a problem, sometimes it feels easier than facing that deep well of hurt that can be found within our souls — a well of unanswered questions. Like, for example, what is this journey about? What am I supposed to do with my time? What's up with the 9-to-5 job thing anyway? Is marriage with the picket fence the answer to where my life is headed? What is next?

So how did I cope? What did I do that helped me change,

make amends, and beat the 'fear jitters' and regain my footing? I realized I didn't like the title of my book and I decided to change the cover design. Yes, metaphorically speaking, of course. But I changed my course. I altered my thoughts. Like Norman Vincent Peale said, "Change your thoughts and change your world."

As a young woman who was always a journal writer, I turned to pen and paper to help me find a change in thinking. This is an exercise you can apply to your own life. It's fun. It's simple and it requires you to spend some time thinking about a very important subject: YOU.

Do you know what the cover of your own book would be? Do you like the title? Do you like where you are on your journey? Is your life headed on the right road? Here is your exercise to apply the story of your life. After all, it's the most important one you will ever read. You may not be physically reading the text, but you are living the actions of your thoughts right now.

So before you change up your scenery just to prove you can, why don't you stay 'still' for a bit and contemplate what you would like Your Story to look like? Take a few moments and do this exercise which you can do in a few minutes, or take a day or a few weeks to do.

Exercise: The Book Title to Your Life

What you will need:

- A blank journal and a pen
- Silence and a creative space that will allow you to tap within to the deeper part of yourself
- An attitude that what you are about to do will actually help set your life on a different course

1. Design the cover—the title with the tagline that describes your journey. Use your favorite book as an example of how to do this. Study the cover and figure out why you love it so much. The

color? The title? The words? What do they reflect? Now apply your own story title to yourself. Write down a few choices and choose one for now so you can complete the exercise. Here is mine:

Be Your Own Rock Star

2. Now write the tagline for the cover title. What is the tagline? This is the one-phrase sentence you will see on the cover of a book that gives you a brief description of why you would want to read it. It is the 'hook' to attract the reader to buy the book. Here is an example of one of my favorite books: *Eat Pray Love* by Elizabeth Gilbert. The tagline to this now-legendary memoir was *One woman's search for everything across Italy, India and Indonesia.* Right away you have a sense of what this book is about. A woman in search of something more in her world. Sounds intriguing. Yes, sign me up. Now what does your tagline look like? Take time and write a few choices. But make sure it's one that resembles the title. This should be a fun space for you to reflect on what you want your own book story to say. How intriguing is it? If you don't currently like the 'tagline,' like I didn't when I was living as a younger girl in Hollywood, *change it!* "It's never too late to become what you might have been"—a quote by the English author George Eliot is fitting here. (Did you know that 'George Eliot' was merely a male 'pen name' for Mary Anne Evans? Mary Anne became a famous English novelist under the assumed identity of being a male to ensure that her works were taken seriously. Sometimes a change in title is just what our own personal world may be needing.) Here is an example of my tagline:

Learn how to be the rock star of your own journey and beat your fears down to a nub

3. Now write the inside jacket if you are imagining a hardcover book. Or if you are thinking paperback, the back-of-the-book description in two compelling paragraphs that speak to your soul personally and can reflect to an outside person just exactly what your quest is, what your purpose is, and what story you are telling with your own personal journey.

Here is mine:

Machel Shull grew up in the Midwest in Southern Missouri. Her country-girl spirit has stayed with her on her quest to enjoy and see life and share her soul with others. From being a model at an early age to becoming a comedic actress in her twenties, Machel thrives on challenge, change and meeting others. She believes in mystical things, Christ, love, hope, faith and being a person that can help others always. In this memoir discover how one young girl left Missouri in search of something greater than four corners of the hayfields that surrounded her childhood memories. With love, faith and mishaps, Machel is hoping to become a true Rock Star of her own story by sharing her vulnerabilities and reaching out to others. Will she find her soul mate? Does she discover what her inner strengths are? And why did she leave Hollywood? Find out inside the pages of her own life story that describes openly her personal story of love, loss, hope and renewal.

The back cover or inside jacket is more of a 'tease' that gives people a little 'food for thought' to entice them to read your story. Yes, this is your life. Can you describe from an outside point of view what you are reflecting? Remember, if you don't like where you are, take this time to write how you want it to change. Just like the young girl who didn't like being the Poor Me type she discovered in *The Celestine Prophecy*, you can change your course and become who you've always wanted to be.

4. Design the chapters. Map them out. Write an outline of what you are hoping your book to be—your life—your story!

Take time to get creative. This can be a sentence or a paragraph long or even a page. Whatever you need to do to make this feel 'real.' Like this story is you, yours, and what you want to show the world. Take time to add or create as much as you need.

5. What is your *decree*? This you can think of as sort of like New Year's resolutions. I like to call it 'my year's decree.' What do I want to happen in this one year? I write it out at the beginning of each year and then read it each month to see if I am on track. I even keep it in a document on my phone so I can read it every so often for inspiration. Not all of what I shoot for happens each year. But I find that over half of my goals and desires materialize because I am actively feeding and suggesting to my mind what I am hoping for. If I haven't met these objectives, I try to kick them into gear before the year is over. Here are my examples:

- Write a book
- Yoga
- Go to church 2–3 times a month
- Keep the house clean
- Be a better wife and mom
- Paint
- Keep running

I don't want to bore you. But you can see they are not some massively significant things that are impossible to accomplish. Make your goals real, and accessible. If they are larger ones that take more time, add this into the chapter section of your life's story.

You are interesting. You are the only person in this world that is you. Discover what you are here for. Take time to like and cultivate your own personal world. Take time to write your book cover. Write your tagline that is compelling and motivates you to stay inspired. Write your inside jacket cover with a few teaser lines that are motivating to your own life story. What do you want to unfold? Add that as a teaser line here. Write your chapters out. Write a yearly 'decree' for yourself.

So you say you are now in your mid-life and your story has changed. Map out the last half. One of the most important things anyone has ever told me came from a woman who was my therapist in Hollywood, Dr Tess Hightower. I was privileged to know her and learn from her. If you read *Middle Age Beauty* then you know that I interviewed Tess in an important chapter about why you should never lie about your age. And she also shared with me an important analogy about life. She used her hands to show me a span of air about 6 feet wide. She showed me that this half of your life has already happened. Then Tess took that half (with her hands) and said, "This half does not have to look like the first half of your life. You can make this half whatever you want to still." (In so many words she said this!)

Well, that was music to my ears. To learn that my first half doesn't have to be my last half and that I can still create and visualize whatever I want. So can you. Don't ever listen to those who try to cast a shadow of fear over your dream. Don't listen to the naysayers. If you lose friends who don't support your current life change, have the courage to build a new bridge, meet new folks who will take you 'higher.'

The world-famous and extraordinary Oprah Winfrey is known for saying, "Surround yourself only with people who are going to *take you higher*." Listen to those words. Believe in a new world that mirrors the story you want to tell with your own life. Don't be afraid to change. Go deep inside. Discover your own greatness. Have the courage to share the real you. Be your own best book title, and don't forget that at any time you can rewrite the story if you start heading down the wrong path. A quote to encompass this is by novelist and writer, Deena Metzger: "When stories nestle in the body, the soul comes forth."

If you let go a little, you will have a little peace. If you let go a lot, you will have a lot of peace. If you let go completely, you will discover complete peace.

~ Achaan Chah

Chapter 28

Non Attachment and Finding a Balance

Life can be a battle of pushing and pulling. Trying to set and attain goals. Making our quotas. Hitting the gym. Watching our calorie intake, putting up with office drama, battling traffic. "When will things go my way? When will it be my turn? Why this? Why that?" Maybe you are one of the lucky ones walking the planet who cannot identify with the pull/push process of life. So if you aren't one of the lucky ones, *what can you do to gain balance?*

Non Attachment

I remember in 2003 when my Zen teacher slid across the table a paragraph from a book regarding the power of 'non attachment,' I quickly read it, processed it, and slid it back and said, "I don't agree with that." (Basically the paragraph stated that non-attachment will help you find inner peace and more happiness.)

Sometimes we are not ready for our lessons or the hard truths we must face that can help us find that much-needed inner peace.

I had been that girl. The one who thought she had it all figured out. I had all my dreams in place. I knew where I belonged in the world. I had my future lined out, too. Well, of course we make plans and you know who laughs. I now look back and realize that I was too young and also not ready to let go of my own attachments—my illusions that gave my soul a certain box to sit in so that I knew my own perimeters. I liked being in this place that allowed me to feel and think exactly the way I could under-stand. This method works for only a little while. Then you will be faced with seeing your own flaws and wondering once again where you went wrong in your thinking.

'Non Attachment.' That doesn't make sense really. Obviously since we were born we were taught to love things, people and places—to feel attachments that define us. So if we are taught this, what is the importance of unlearning it?

For me personally, I still struggle with this. You know, I get my hopes up about something. A situation, or an event that may come to pass. I decorate this event with Christmas tree trimmings. I see the lights, I put my heart and soul into this 'idea,' and then I count down to when that moment might happen. What we want sometimes just doesn't happen. That particular event unravels. Or worse, that person we wanted to reciprocate our feelings doesn't. When this happens, the most crippling feelings can drag us down and make us feel as if…well, "Why dream? What is this life? When is it my turn?"

Why get excited about something if there is a possibility it might not work out?

For me, I have found a sort of in-between balance of non attachment and the realism of how I was raised that keeps me grounded just enough and also keeps my feet slightly lifted off the earth. I reach up to the sky so I can keep believing anyway when my heart aches from a disappointment.

These lessons teach me (us) to go deeper. They teach us to find out what might be missing from our internal world that needs attention. When you seek to fill a void with something else, there is almost a guaranteed certainty that you will be disappointed.

So find a balance between your hopes and non attachment. There is an in-between place that we can access where our souls can fly, find peace and still believe in our dreams.

Elegance is being equally beautiful inside and out.
~ Coco Chanel

Chapter 29

Why Appearance Matters to Your Soul

What does it feel like to be over the age of 40? Honestly, these last two years have been two of the best years in my life. The beginnings of this book materialized from my own personal struggles and victories as a woman who has been associated first with her looks, before her spirit. Being a model and acting part time for a few years in Hollywood truly added an insightful perspective on the importance of your appearance.

Now some may argue that placing importance on how someone looks is considered shallow. However, whether we like it or not, society does judge us by the way we look. Our appearance is one of the most important assets or hindrances we face when coming to the workforce. According to an article posted in the *Wall Street Journal*, written by Sue Shellenbarger, "Attractive people are likely to earn an average of 3% to 4% more than a person with below-average looks. That adds up to $230,000 more over a lifetime for the typical good-looking person."

Forget about that fact. Take care of your appearance to signal to your soul that you care about YOU.

Are you taking time to make yourself look the best you can each day?

This is something you should consider. Don't just run around in sweats because that feels more comfortable, even if you are a stay-at-home mom. Take time to apply your make-up, wear some perfume and paint your nails. Take time to do your hair. Develop a routine that will allow you to make time for yourself in the morning.

You don't have to be a beauty queen in order to look great. Your appearance and how you want to present yourself to the world should be something you seriously consider. If you want to think that what you look like and wear does not reflect the real you, you are seriously wrong. World-renowned French designer Coco Chanel left us with many indelible quotes that we should remember. Two quotes that fit perfectly here are: "A woman who doesn't wear perfume has no future," and "Dress shabbily and they remember the dress; dress impeccably and they remember the woman." Are you taking time to consider your appearance?

You should. Let me share with you some of my own ups and downs with my appearance. I went through a 'bohemian poet' period during the middle of my twenties. After being a model and under intense scrutiny on a weekly basis, I converted to long sweaters and skirts and Sinead O'Connor hiking boots. During this phase I looked more like a potato sack and nothing like myself. As I revolted about beauty and the emphasis on beauty, I found myself becoming more reclusive, introspective and less joyful.

For whatever reason, I happen to be particularly affected by the clothes I choose to wear. During this sabbatical from attracting energy from the way I dressed, I also began to lose money during my bookings. Why? I stopped booking commercials. I stopped looking like my fabulous self and was trying to get society to take me seriously and look at me for my brain. What I realized and learned was that I consciously altered my appearance to try and change an attitude toward my outward appearance. Afraid that I might be labeled as an 'airhead' because I was blonde, I turned off my 'light' and went into hiding under hideous clothes and long skirts. I cut my hair. I wore my reading glasses when I honestly couldn't see with them on. I wanted the world to take me seriously and not as just another blonde in Hollywood. My soul felt so little and frightened. I was giving my inner self mixed signals. Soon, I had intervention with my manager at the time. She confronted me and asked me, "Why are just your hands showing? You are covered from head to toe!"

Uhh, I had to think about that. I did. Why had I gone to such an extreme? Where had my sparkle gone? I hadn't gone completely Gothic, but I was headed down that path.

My X Factor had been smeared by my casual appearance.

Well, luckily for me, I was someone who worked well with constructive criticism. I managed to listen and do some inner investigating on why I had gone down this path. I discovered during this period of my life that my appearance did indeed influence my mood and sense of well-being. Of course there were trying times later when I entered motherhood and I thought being glamorous was something of the past because I was a mother. But that does not have to be the case. Now I don't mean you have to look like Zsa Zsa Gabor every day, but there is no reason not to try to look as pretty as possible.

If you are single, you never know what man might be lurking just around the corner. The next time you run to Starbucks for a quick jolt, don't just throw on your flip flops and your comfortable sweats. Take 15 minutes to beautify your own natural appearance.

Maybe it's a necklace and earrings. Maybe it's just a fabulous jacket. The trick is to at least make an effort. You don't want to lose that right guy to the wrong girl because one day you were too lazy to feel and look your best.

The world can indeed be a cruel place. So make the most of your natural looks.

Try to coordinate a style that will help you exude confidence. Be bold. Remember Coco Chanel's words. *Leave an impression that represents your best You.*

I may no longer be a model. I am no longer an actress. I am just a woman in her forties who is a wife and a mother living in the suburbs in Southern California. But you can bet that when I leave the house, I take a few moments to myself to improve my mood by investing a few minutes in my personal appearance because...why?

Because it's good to care enough about my outward appearance so I can signal to my inner self that I care about me. I like me. I am worth looking good for, each day.

Here are just a few simple tips that can help you feel more like a pin-up queen:

- Wear lipstick every day. Maybe it's a nude lip gloss that's more natural. The trick is to give your face a little love and cheer up the corners a bit.
- Always wear a touch of perfume. Find your signature scent and wear it always.
- Never leave the house without some make-up. Maybe you have that sculpted face with the arched eyebrows and perfect pouty lips. If so, maybe you can disregard this request. But for me, with my blonde hair, fair skin and naked brows, nothing is more tiring than hearing, "Are you not feeling well today? Are you tired?" No, I just happen to be one of those women who do sparkle with a little more make-up. Nothing wrong with that. The trick is to know if you do or not. You be the judge.
- Always make sure your nails and toes are painted with a brilliant color. Reds, mauves and dark pinks are my personal favorites. My sister personally loves that French manicure. Her nails are always perfect. Take time to observe how many times a day you look at your hands. If your nail polish is chipped or worn down to the nub, there is a good possibility this feeling will silently tap away at

your confidence all day.

- Always style your hair. Do you like a ponytail? Do you enjoy the straight look like all the *Friends* sitcom girls? Take time to do a hairdo before you leave the house.
- Invest in stylish jackets and long coats that can just glam up any pair of jeans or black pair of leggings. I happen to frequent some upscale consignment shops to find my coats. Audrey Hepburn is of course my inspiration. Don't forget to find your own Icon who inspires you to look fabulous.
- Find one name brand that you feel personifies your looks. Is it Donna Karan, Ralph Lauren, or do you love bright colors like Lily Pulitzer? Find one brand and coordinate it accordingly into your daily lifestyle.
- Spend no less than 10–15 minutes (this is pretty fast!) on polishing your appearance like a sparkling diamond. Don't forget, Mr Right or an unexpected opportunity could be happening today! Be prepared with your best outfit.

Don't forget Johann Friedrich von Schiller's permeating words: "Appearance rules the world." Even if you don't agree with those four words, what if you happen to be wrong? Take my advice and don't chance it! Look fabulous. Seize today and make this your moment in the sun. Life is too short to let all the glamour queens in the magazines have all the fun. Don't miss a golden moment because you forgot to wear your lipstick!

Okay, I confess. I do struggle with this. I have to force myself out of my comfy clothes and into that outfit that makes my soul feel a bit more on fire. If it weren't for my husband I might have easily become one of those I-am-a-granola-girl-therefore-fashion-does-not-apply-to-me types. And if the granola type makes your soul sing, well go for that look then. Remember Mark Twain's quote, "Be casual in your dress if you must, but keep a tidy soul." Only you can figure out how you feel best in what kind of wardrobe you wear, but how your soul feels on the inside is always the most important thing. I would like to point out though, "if you must" is the key phrase in Mark Twain's quote. I do believe he was a man that wore suits...at least in his distinguishing photos. "Clothes make the Man"—he was quoted saying that, too. Maybe he was onto something. So remember to take care of your outer appearance and watch the inner *you* light up a little.

Not all Heroes wear capes and tight pants. Mine has a violin and wears poofy skirts.
~ From a Lindsey Stirling fan

Chapter 30

Interview — with Rock Star Violinist, Lindsey Stirling

I sat in four hours' worth of rush-hour traffic to see Lindsey Stirling one beautiful spring day.

The traffic to Los Angeles from San Diego looked more like parked cars at a shopping mall. I had no way around it though. My son's birthday party wish was taking his best friend with him up to see a violinist at the Henry Fonda Theatre named Lindsey Stirling. I had no idea that I, too, was just about to witness 'greatness' before my very eyes. Sometimes we don't know when a blessing is right around the corner.

When Lindsey came out onto the stage, I knew something special was about to happen when I witnessed the crowd's pre-show excitement of just anticipating that big moment when she first stepped out onto the stage.

When the lights went down, and Lindsey came out, the next two hours were just an incredible, inspirational ride of music, joy and stories from Lindsey. She shared about going to a poor country in Africa and how the kids in the tribe were just so excited to have a toothbrush. She shared with her fans her gratitude for being so supportive and showing up to her concerts all over the world. She shared with us how her dream did not die on a talent competition show just because the judges couldn't figure out where she would fit in as a musician/composer/rocker/dancer/solo violinist.

Turns out they were right. Lindsey Stirling didn't fit. She actually created a new form of music that forged fans all over the world...like my son and others that loved her videos and music so much. What I witnessed that night touched my heart and soul.

After I got home that night, I told my husband how much I loved Lindsey Stirling and he said, "You should try and interview her for your 'Soul' book."

A few months later, you can only imagine my incredible delight, that I am able to share with you HER story in her own words. I have said too much. My words are not important here. Let Lindsey tell the story:

Lindsey, seeing your concert at the Henry Fonda Theatre was one of my top inspirational moments of 2013. Your performance and your message inspired not only me, but everyone there from all age groups. What encouraging words could you share on how to follow dreams without compromising spirit?

Lindsey Stirling: I think there are definitely forces among us for good and forces that are not. Ultimately, we have to decide where we stand, what our beliefs are, and what we are and are not willing to do before we get put into that situation where we have to choose. When I am pressured to make a choice, especially where my morals are concerned, it is easier to do the right thing when I have really already made that decision a long time ago. The bottom line is that if you don't know where you stand it will be very easy for others to use you, manipulate you, and pressure you into doing things you might later regret. I know that as I pursue my dreams I have to constantly remind myself of why I started my journey in the first place and not allow myself to get lost in the process.

What I loved about your musical performance was also how you interacted with the crowd. You spoke inspiring words to build up each person there on the value of staying true to yourself and pursuing your dreams. Can you give an example that defined your own courage when you prevailed

because you chose to live a soulful journey by following your own heart? What happened after that? Were you surprised by the results of how 'staying true to yourself' was exactly what attracted so many devoted fans and those who admire your music?

Lindsey Stirling: From the very beginning it was very important to me not only to succeed, but to show the world that I could do so on my own terms and without compromising myself or my standards. I wanted to be an example and prove that it could be done. Little did I know how difficult that was going to be, ha ha! I was given several promising opportunities that were extremely tempting; opportunities that I had to turn down. For example, during my first year after *America's Got Talent*, a popular mainstream artist wanted to collaborate with me and I was absolutely thrilled! But once I heard the lyrics of the song I was supposed to cover and I started looking at their album, I realized that the music wasn't something I could support. Not only did I have to tell them "no thanks" after having already told them "yes" (super-awkward!), I also started feeling discouraged. I began thinking that, maybe, in order to be a popular artist I really would have to compromise some things...and that was something I was unwilling to do. But I have never been one to give up easily! I kept working and praying and moving forward. That same year I released "Crystallize," and it changed everything.* To say I was surprised by its success would be an understatement, ha ha, but it felt amazing to have succeeded despite the odds, and without compromising myself in the process.

In 2011, you reached over 400 million views and 3 million subscribers to your videos on YouTube, then went on to sell out worldwide in concert in 2013. The accolades continue...

How did that feel? Do you think your commitment to your soul, and your courage to keep your vision, is what took you the distance and still is today?

Lindsey Stirling: When I started pursuing a career in music I did so with the attitude that "If I am meant to do this, God will help make it happen. If I'm not, then I guess I'll find out." Ha ha. I wanted it so badly and I really felt like my Heavenly Father wanted me to succeed too. After *America's Got Talent*, I was simply devastated because I had felt so strongly that I was inspired to compete and that my Heavenly Father had wanted me to do well. I didn't realize it at that time, but He had other plans for me, and I just needed to be patient, move forward, and find out what those plans were. I really believe that I have been given the opportunity to tour the world and share my music because I have a message to share. I love interacting with people and I want to empower and inspire and make this world a better place. I suppose that ultimately it is love—love for others, love of music, love of God, love of myself—that has gotten me to this point.

If you could give one message to someone reading this who could be at a 'crossroads' and feel like they want to quit because fear has set in or their critics say it's impossible, what would you tell them on why they must not give up?

Lindsey Stirling: It is those moments of despair, when we think that all is lost and that we should just give up, that make or break us. Do we try again, do we open a new door, do we push forward with faith? Or do we let the pressures of life crush our resolve? Looking back on my life, it was during those times when I felt like giving up that I had almost succeeded. I think that if it were possible for us to see into the future—if we could see what would happen to us if we didn't give up—we wouldn't.

I also noticed how you shared so much sincere gratitude with your fans. Do you think that gratitude is a key element to being more soulful? Do you think that has been a catalyst to your sell-out concerts and devoted fan base because you seem to share an 'open heart' with them on stage?

Lindsey Stirling: I believe that sincere gratitude is the key to happiness. When I visited Kenya, I was expecting to see the typified poverty we often see of Africa on the news. However, the people I saw were some of the happiest, healthiest, most beautiful people I had ever met.* I asked myself how they could be so happy when they had so little—by most world standards they were very poor. But these people were so grateful for the little they had. I realized that I didn't need material possessions or fame or the perfect house or the perfect job to be happy. I could choose to be happy by appreciating what I already had. I am indeed extremely grateful to my fans all over the world who have listened to my music, bought my album, come to my concerts…it's all so humbling and I feel so very honored that they are willing to take part in this epic journey with me.

What do you do to enrich your spirit and bring fulfillment to your personal life?

Lindsey Stirling: Honestly I love what I do for a living, and I feel very blessed to say that almost everything I get to do as part of that (performing, making videos, creating music, interacting with people) is extremely fulfilling. My work is my play. But when I'm not 'working,' I love spending time with my family and friends back at home. I can usually convince them to do silly random things with me (makes for *great* videos, ha ha).* I love playing board games with my family. I love ice cream. And on rare occasions I enjoy a good movie.

I find it absolutely wonderful that you are inspiring teenagers to listen to classical music in a new genre that you basically created with your music. Your violin music is not only uplifting but bringing teenagers (and all ages!) to follow an important musical genre, which they might have missed out on if it weren't for your talent, courage and gumption. What advice would you give to them on how developing a passion for what they love can add so much more enjoyment to their lives?

Lindsey Stirling: Don't live life in a box. I am, of course, extremely supportive of education in all its forms, but I think that society generally has a cookie-cutter idea of what education is, and that goes for music too. I almost gave up on violin because I was getting tired of performing other composers' classical music day in and day out, year after year. I'm not saying that we shouldn't learn from the great masters of the past (we should), but I think that the desire to create, in one form or another, is ingrained deep within each of us, and that our greatest joy comes when we create something original…something that says, "I exist for a reason and I have something to say!"

How has *your* passion for music grounded *you* and given *you* soul wings to fly?

Lindsey Stirling: I feel like the music I create is an extension of me. The *fantastic* thing about music is that it has the ability to communicate without words. There is something divine about it…and it has a way of extracting beauty from within us.

I have often found a greater understanding of myself through the music I create. Not only has the creation process been liberating for me, but creating music has also given me the freedom to live my dreams.

* Lindsey Stirling videos:
"Crystallize":
http://www.youtube.com/watch?v=aHjpOzsQ9YI

Africa:
http://www.youtube.com/watch?v=0g9poWKKpbU

Fun with family and friends:
http://www.youtube.com/watch?v=R_clIrMfUTM
http://www.youtube.com/watch?v=zd02XlpiEvM

Joy can spring like a flower even from the cliffs of despair.
~ Anne Morrow Lindbergh

Chapter 31

Grief and Pain—How Do We Carry On?

Sometimes we must endure change in order to discover the simple beauty around us. We may be too busy or think that happiness is something 'out there' worth trying to attain. At our fingertips are a few simple tasks, tricks and actions that can transform our daily lives with moments of bliss.

I will begin by sharing with you a personal story of a delightful chapter in my life. Isn't it wonderful when you have a cherished group of friends? During my mid-thirties when I worked full time as an advertising executive for a couple of newspapers in Southern California, I had this marvelous core group of friends who would meet weekly at a place that felt like our own "Cheers" in Rancho Santa Fe. Friday night we would sit together over a few drinks as the piano man played his various upbeat tunes and life spilled out and around us in the most delicious way so that one had the feeling those days would never end. That this romantic period of love and good times with a close-knit group would be here in the future. Such are wishful thoughts that you do not recognize when you are having them because you believe them, because what you feel is all you can see and believe in...you know, the 'now' of those moments.

This wonderful time period lasted for about two to three years, I think, when I look back. I would host mini-celebrations late into the evening with my fiancé at the time (my husband now) and his friends, too. We shared our dreams, we toasted our thoughts, and we felt romantic, young and full of life. We walked around in a haze of happy times, centered around a cocktail or two that always made the evening more like a technical moment in Hollywood.

I thought this magical phase of whimsy, carefree living with my buddies would continue... That's just what we are always hoping in life. When the good is great, please stay on course, shall we? However, sometimes, just like in a poignant novel, we do not always see the signs that may allow us to see change on the horizon.

We discover sometimes that those we love can leave us. That what we enjoy doing can sometimes fade. Our careers can falter. We may trip on our own mistakes or be too close to the circumstances to see something obvious that is right in front of our eyes. We are having too much fun to realize that it's just about to end...

I remember my husband and I wondered why the phone stopped ringing when we were first married. Instead of being the couple who would be getting married, we had quickly become a 'married couple,' and our single friends weren't quite as interested in that. During this more introspective period I began to find my love for reading. I began to find some light inside novels by various authors. With more time to be reflective and less being social with my friends, I somehow found great comfort in books.

Just when I thought most changes were done and I was easing into the quietness of married life, I lost a friend to pancreatic cancer at the age of 37. Then something even more earth-shattering happened. I lost a great friend to suicide (I mention this in a chapter in the Love section). The deep feeling of anguish and grief literally knocked me sideways.

The next year marked the beginning of a new decade for me. I just couldn't believe that my friend wouldn't be on the planet that year. Losing his presence and my girlfriend who had died, too—all within a span of six months—took me down a darker path than I had been before. I managed to regain my light slowly but surely. And what about that group of friends who always met for those romantic evenings of intriguing talks and celebrations late into the night? Death separated us all.

Scarred with open wounds by openly grieving for the same person, we all retreated quietly into our own worlds without discussing the hurt and the loss. To see one of those friends during this period was a constant reminder of the pain that cut like a knife, of the loss we had all endured.

I began to do my own research on suicide. I found out some disturbing numbers and alarming figures. According to one mental health prevention site, suicide has increased by 60% over the last 45 years. Every 16 minutes someone is committing suicide in the United States. Worldwide, you can figure every 40 seconds. One year after my friend's death, I participated in a suicide walk with some other friends. When I showed up at the park there were others who had suffered the same fate as I had— a grieving individual left to figure out the pieces of suicide's meaning. I was surprised by the thousands of others there, too.

That day I walked with my friends under the bright sun and remembered a friend who shouldn't have died. I remembered with great nostalgia those few years of our fun times and dreams that seemed like they would never die. I remembered the laughter and the moments that will be etched in my mind always. What is wonderful about life—grief really does heal with time. There are moments when you think that this pain will never go away. The loss is so great, how can we go on?

With much loss, hurt and dramatic shifting, can come clarity and reconciliation to what really matters most. During the next few years I found myself actively seeking to live a more present life by living in 'now' moments instead of in the past or the future. I prayed more. I found more gratitude and I actively sought ways to cultivate a more mindful, deep-seated existence that was grounded in the action of 'small joys' and counting my blessings.

I miss that time that seemed to go on forever with that kind of carefree joy you think can last. I miss those friends who gathered around the piano bar and found joy in sharing the moments with one another. I miss that golden age of believing time would not end. That there would not need to be another beginning.

Albert Camus once wrote:

In the depths of winter, I finally learned that within me there lay an invincible summer.

Life can be brutal. So the trick is to find some simple actions, tricks and lessons we can apply in our daily lives that can help us weather any storm. I am now learning to still have fun with new friends and with loved ones, but most importantly, with *myself*. Life can bring us joy, sorrow, and love. How we navigate through the unfolding of each moment of change can sometimes be the most important lesson of all.

A genuine odyssey is not about piling up experiences. It is a deeply felt, risky and unpredictable tour of the soul.
~ Thomas Moore

Chapter 32

Quiet Time for the Soul—Even If It Lands on Your Birthday

Today is my 43rd birthday. I think that I shall share with you the honest truth of pain, love and loss. This book is called *Live Love Soul*. But in order to be happy, one must examine one's life, understand one's own soul, and be willing to overturn the rocks in the big open field of our mind to find out what is under those hidden places we wish to pretend do not exist.

I shall just tell you that today I did not wake up bursting with joy—"Wow! Yay! I am alive!" It doesn't always happen like that as we know. Sometimes there is an ache in our soul that calls us back, pulls us in to look for something deeper or to find out what is missing. Some may run from this feeling. Or just keep on with their merry routine of busyness so they don't need to reflect on what the ache could be in their own heart.

I do just the opposite. I face it. I sit with it. I want to understand it. I feel the feeling that might even be painful so I can learn from this moment. It is easy to understand why my birthday isn't such a joyous occasion as it used to be. I had previously, for many years, celebrated—big fat celebrations with tequila shots, party hats and dancing on the tables—with a crowd of friends, acquaintances, loved ones at a lovely restaurant nestled in the town of Rancho Santa Fe. For six years straight this was it. For a woman of only 43 (yes, sort of a joke, but then not!) this is a good stretch of regularity. This celebration, place, friends and repetition all had such a loving spirit wrapped around it that filled my birthday each year with verve, fun, laughs and importance.

This year I had arranged a tea with a new friend and my cherished mentor. We were to sit and eat finger sandwiches together and sip tea out of fine china with pink roses near the ocean. But as the days crept closer to my birthday, an eerie feeling of sadness just sat on me, begging me to stay quiet—alone instead.

I so did not want this to be my day. You know. In my pajamas drinking coffee and writing about my friend who committed suicide. But in order to write this book from a loving place with an open smile of intent and joy, I find it only fair to share with you: I have wounds, too. I hurt, too. Life is not always perfect. There will be a day when something unexpected or crushing can happen. We never saw it coming. There were no warning signs. Nothing to tell us to hold on, *watch out*, the rug is about to come out from under you and your life will never be the same.

Well, that happened to me. In one fell swoop. The joy was knocked out of me that year. One must understand the ebb and flow of life. That with great joy there will be sadness. With great love there can be pain. And as I write about meditating and quieting the soul, I also learn that the soul has a place of rest that it needs. A moment to recharge, to refuel. To feel sad or reflective if necessary in order to gain clarity about the past.

I look back over the years and I see myself with a wide-open heart not knowing the rawness of this life. The pain that can instill great intense jagged jabs of hurt in the dark alone in the night. I see a girl who had a party hat on and just wanted to have fun. And celebrate, because isn't that what life is about?

No.

Life is our journey that I have found we need to learn from as well. This life is ours to find solace and grace. This life is ours to figure out why there might be that dull ache calling us to look back—take a deep look to understand that what remains can still heal with each passing day.

So instead, this morning on my 43rd birthday, I enjoyed a small ritual of love with the birds outside early in the morning. I watched them in their beauty, their sweet music and flight of grace. I watched my red Doberman in our little backyard fenced in by a hill in a small beach town observe these birds, too. I drank my coffee with just a little bit of cinnamon and half-and-half. I thought about the brisk morning air and how refreshing it felt to breathe outside beauty in. I sat there in my pink T-shirt and brown baggy cut-off sweats, okay with the fact I had taken time for myself and then thought about this:

Today is my birthday and it's okay if I am not with friends. It's okay if I don't wear a mask in the charade of trying to make my life grand. Sometimes life can be more grand if I just sit, watch, observe and learn from the nature around me. I need this quiet space today. I need to relax alone, write, read, cuddle up with my favorite book and just observe these feelings.

Tonight I will be enjoying the evening with my son and my husband. We will be taking a little drive to Pauma Valley where my in-laws own a ranch. There we will play a game of Monopoly, eat some Mexican food and just be cozy. No big parties. I shall remember and find joy. I shall sit quietly today with my soul and count my blessings. Life is truly in the here and now. The trick is to stay in tune with your soul. That voice that beckons to be heard. You need to nourish the inner you that needs to be loved.

Find seeds of hope. Go within. Keep rekindling the innocence we had as a child. Have faith in the good and in a loving world. We must make an effort to be a Live Love Soul. Happiness is something that can be achieved by the smallest act of just petting your cat. It can be found in monitoring the sky of changing clouds. Happiness is not *out there* waiting to be had. It is within *you* to make for yourself. So if you wake up one day and don't feel joyful, take time to recognize why. Do some internal searching. Find out what your soul needs to be fed. Maybe it could just be a little quiet time alone so you can hear your thoughts. Your soul needs some quiet time to heal to recharge. To

remember, to be grateful, to find peace with what has been lost...
So make quiet time for yourself, even if it happens to be a
birthday.

Today I am 43 years old. I am making a quiet space to talk to
you, dear reader, to tell you, yes this life can hurt, but there is so
much to live for, so much to discover and to be, still. And even
after we lose those we love, there is still more to unearth, to
create, to make and to share. There could be a new person around
the corner who will feel like an angel of cheer—a new friend who
just loves you unconditionally. Believe in the good. Believe in
your chance to be happy. Out of the mystery of life new worlds
are created. What we cannot see is there just slightly out of reach.
So reach for it, dear readers! I wish you much peace and love. I wish
you to find a quiet space to retreat to, so you can learn more
about yourself. The great philosopher Socrates boldly stated,
"The unexamined life is not worth living." He felt that we must
go within to find out more about ourselves...

So remember to throw off your party hats. Get down to the
basics. Get down on your knees and do some internal searching.
Pull out those weeds. Do your hard work on yourself so you can
grow. Even if this means on your birthday to cancel a tea party,
by all means give your soul the little quiet time it deserves. Your
real friends, the ones who truly love you, will understand...*mine
did*.

Believe in yourself! Have faith in your abilities! Without a humble but reasonable confidence in your own powers you cannot be successful or happy.
~ Norman Vincent Peale

Chapter 33

Interview—with Dr Doris Lee McCoy on the Search for Happiness

I met Dr Doris Lee McCoy during my newspaper columnist days in Rancho Santa Fe. I was always looking for a story to share or someone to feature in my column. I met her at a fancy restaurant under the eucalyptus trees in this affluent town. Soon we were sharing our stories (the power of a story!) and I was enthralled by Dr Doris's larger-than-life attitude on positivity. Her attitude was reminiscent of my favorite philosopher, Norman Vincent Peale. And, yes, I am aware that I have already mentioned him before now. I am just giving you a gauge of Dr Doris's 'positive thinking style.' Her attitude and writing is rooted much deeper than the current millennium's Internet searches for research on topics and looking for a new meme to make us laugh. Dr Doris has traveled the world and interviewed prestigious dignitaries and searched high and low for what brings happiness on a 'whole' to a community. And where on earth is the happiest place in the world?

Dr Doris was kind enough to share her findings here with me and you. She is a true Rock Star and a woman I so admire. Thank you, Dr Doris, for adding your words to this book.

Here is my interview with Dr Doris Lee McCoy:

Doris, you have accomplished so much and find so much enthusiasm in how you perceive life. This is all exemplified through the books you write and the people you interview. What common factor have you noticed out of your 3000 interviews with 'visionaries' of our time? Do you see a correlation between their well-being and success?

Dr Doris Lee McCoy: I believe the common factors would be:

1. They all had great passion for what they were doing.
2. They used negative experiences to discover their strengths and grow into better people.
3. They developed their self-esteem and a positive attitude.
4. They become more decisive and disciplined, set goals and reach them.
5. Their actions reflect their integrity and they encourage others to win.
6. They are persistent with everything that they do.
7. They take more risks.
8. They hone their communication and problem-solving skills.
9. They surround themselves with competent, responsible, supportive people.
10. They schedule time for exercise and recreation, plus stay healthy.
11. They keep their faith.
12. They are making a contribution to whatever is most meaningful to them.

What advice would you give to your readers who struggle with depression and are looking for daily methods to help change their attitude, while bringing their confidence level up, too?

Dr Doris Lee McCoy: 'Learning by Doing' should bring you partially out of depression. Doing something that is constructive will show you right away that you are able to accomplish something new.

In your book, *Gross National Happiness*, you share how 'happiness' can be measured by the cities and geography of

where individuals lived. Which one was number one and could you explain why?

Dr Doris Lee McCoy: There are a variety of different lists, but the one that I found to be most reliable was the one that was done outside of England. So, Denmark was the number one, followed by Sweden, Switzerland, Austria, Norway, Finland, and Bhutan. Denmark, which was number one, and the rest that follow, are run by socialistic governments, which means that all people are taken care of. The amazing thing about Bhutan being eighth: each person only makes $1,150 a year, and yet they still feel that their country is the happiest place on earth. So money, for them, is not the deciding factor of happiness.

Do you see a direct correlation between positive thinking and the outcome for someone who has achieved their aspirations and dreams? How do you stay so upbeat and positive each day?

Dr Doris Lee McCoy: I certainly do see a correlation between positive thinking and achieving goals. That does not necessarily mean that everything that person wanted in life was completely fulfilled; however, they stay positive. As for myself, one way to stay upbeat is to spend a few minutes at the end of the day to remind yourself of all the things you have accomplished and all that you want to achieve tomorrow that will help you achieve your goals and be happy.

What is the most important factor in the reader's equation for happiness and why should the reader be striving for their right to be happy?

Dr Doris Lee McCoy: Happiness is an important trait that enables other people to learn from you or see your approach to life and how they too can attain a positive attitude. Being grateful for what it is you do have, and possibly making lists of what those things are, is a big part of the equation, enabling you to see in black and white what you have and what others can use as an example to be happy.

Any last parting words of advice that you would like to share with someone reading this book who is learning to cultivate true 'soul' happiness from the inside out?

Dr Doris Lee McCoy: You first have to see what happiness means to YOU, down in your soul. Is this a journey, not necessarily the final goal? Searching within yourself will make you aware that reaching many of your goals will lead you to your true happiness. Happiness is the secondary spin-off of what we were able to accomplish in our lives. The way we respond will be something that comes from the internal, and will be obvious to others who see us. It does not mean that every day we are extremely happy and pleased with what goes on, but we have enough knowledge and foresight to change things that we are able to change and move towards our soul's true intent.

Love yourself first and everything else falls into line. You really have to love yourself to get anything done in this world.
~ Lucille Ball

Chapter 34

Get Happy by Loving Yourself. You Are a Rock Star

Let's get down to the nitty-gritty. It's time to shape up and ship out that negative critic that looms in your head. You know the one that tells you, "Who do you think you are?" Or, like Muriel in the movie *Muriel's Wedding*, while gazing at the stars, "Sometimes I think I am nothing."

Oh, the let-down. The pain of the small voice that creeps up on us in the dark wee hours of the morning preying on our soul, 'berating us with self-deprecating thoughts' that can take us down the dark well of despair. That voice *needs to be silenced*. It's time to silence your inner critic with a little thought, action and spirit. You need to love that self of yours to make your life happy. And being a 'critical person' to yourself can only set you back and rob you of the daily joy you deserve.

So let's get busy and figure out some easy ways to quiet our minds. Let's be kind to our souls and build our inner being *up* so we feel like *rock stars*.

Yes, you too, can be a Rock Star in your own life. You just need to back off from the criticism a bit.

Give yourself a hug and be sweet to your inner soul. If you are nice to you, you will in turn be 'nicer' to others. Your spirit will feel lighter and your heart will be less burdened.

Now how can we silence the voice? I have a few devices that you can apply that I have learned from other great teachers that work wonders. You will receive immediate effects. Your critic will wonder when Elvis left the building while you weren't looking. You soul will soar with power. And your eyes will glow with confidence.

What you will be doing to silence the inner critic:

- Affirmations
- Meditations
- Memorizing scriptures from the Bible (or positive mantra quotes that you love)
- Quiet moments on the floor. Yes! Grab that yoga mat. The time is now. Or roll out that pretty pink towel so you can make some quiet time to reflect and write out affirmations in your journal. You could even write them on sticky notes so you can see them by your coffee maker or on the front of your refrigerator.

Learn to recognize the cycle so you can stop it before it goes into full swing. How do you do this? By monitoring your bad thoughts and learning to replace them with positive thoughts.

Take this moment right now and write out this simple thought:

I am enough right now. I love Me! I am a brilliant soul who is here for a reason. I am here to make the world a better place. I add something truly amazing to this existence. I am not just here for me. I have a purpose.

I will work today on making one thing better in my life.

Please write here your own personal affirmation that you may need right now on your journey:

This chapter is short because it requires you to do some work. You need to fill your mind and your surroundings with positive seeds of influence that can help you become a happier person by shutting out that negative inner critic that wants to keep you small and cozy. In order to grow and learn new experiences, we may have to stand naked in the early morning light. We must face our inner brilliance and what *we could become* if we had the courage to take action, believe in ourselves, and make our world a place that resembles a Happy Soul.

So get off that couch. Get motivated. Find your happy dance and become the own Rock Star in your story. You deserve to shine in the spotlight just like the next person. There is room for one more star waiting to shine. So work on each day, whittling away that inner critic.

You. Deserve. To. Be. Your. Own. Rock Star.

Go on, give Bono a run for his money. I am sure he would give you a wink and a nod. A rock star to me, after all, is a person just like you or me. We can become that person on our own stage, living the dream. (This might not include a world tour though, since I can't even sing well enough for Karaoke night.)

Life is difficult. This is a great truth, one of the greatest truths. It is a great truth because once we truly see this truth, we transcend it. Once we truly know that life is difficult—once we truly understand and accept it—then life is no longer difficult. Because once it is accepted, the fact that life is difficult no longer matters.
~ M. Scott Peck, *The Road Less Travelled*

Chapter 35

The Soul Kit. Three Little Things You Need for a Rainy Day

I am sure you are one of those individuals who never stumbles. Never has any ups and downs or is never leveled by unforeseen circumstances. If this is you, maybe you can skip the Soul Kit chapter. If you never get knocked down, feel lonely or lose someone you love, this might not apply to you.

You may be one of those who just happen to find the right speed, right temperature, right friends, right circumstances, and you are never knocked off balance. I am hoping by that last sentence you might sense that I am half kidding here. Whether we like it or not, none of us are invincible. We cannot always win the 'great fight in life' we might be fighting, and someone we love might just die before we expected. There are many unforeseen circumstances that can spring forth without us ever seeing them coming.

My most shocking year to date was in 2010 when I lost one 37-year-old girlfriend to pancreatic cancer, then six months later, my good friend committed suicide. You might imagine that two funerals of close friends both dying under the age of 40 sent shockwaves through my universe. Where I had once been a fun-loving, spirited woman, these few months left me silent and vulnerable. I had to retreat to the comfort of 'the little sure things' I could count on. Sometimes something tangible, like a security blanket for a baby, can help soothe our inner wounded soul that needs protecting. You know, something you can reach for, feel, touch, and is accessible in your daily life. This is not a person. No, this Soul Kit will be tangible objects that you can hold onto for when the times get rough and you need guidance and inspiration.

I have used each of these tangible things through hardships. I know they will still be there in the future when the unforeseen can happen. You must prepare yourself with a little shield of armor that can help your soul feel grounded. Especially if your foundation is crumbling underneath you or you are going through life-shifting changes that can be scary or cause fear.

Soul Kit List

1. Prayer box

During my mid-twenties I lived on my own before smartphones and the Internet. The closest thing to technology in my little guesthouse in Studio City was a VCR player and a collection of old movies. I could add an answering machine. That was the thing you lived for when you were single: "You have three messages." Sometimes on the weekend it might say, "You have no messages." The fear of a Friday night alone in Hollywood. Oh, I had friends. I had hang-outs. But sometimes it was just easier to stay in and do some soul work. It was during this time that I read about a 'prayer box.' I think it might have been in *Guideposts Magazine*. I am not sure now, as I recall, how this one originated. But what I can tell you is what that little prayer box did for me:

- Peace
- Comfort
- Security

I had been given a gift from Tiffany's jewelry store from a friend. So I had this perfect little turquoise box that I emptied out and then handwrote a little note on top that said "Prayer Box" across the Tiffany label. I am sure any other little cardboard box would work. You might try a craft store or even an office supply store for one that you could use. Then write that little creed on top and place it somewhere you can see every day. I placed mine on my bedside table. Then, on a night when that inner voice of fear might creep in on me, like that lonely Friday night feeling, I would sit at my table and write out little wishes and prayers. I would then take my scissors and cut these prayers into little strips of paper and fold them up and tuck them inside the box.

I remember the prayer box becoming rather cluttered with prayers and wishes, when one day, one was answered, and I felt so excited! I then divided the box into two separate areas with a tissue paper dividing the 'prayers still in waiting' and the 'answered prayers' tucked underneath the tissue. After a year, you could imagine the sweet feeling of security this tangible little box gave me next to my bed. Inside were prayers that were answered and ones 'still existing' in my world. A prayer or wish box can help you maintain what you are wanting to happen in your life and can also help you gauge what your soul is needing. So taking time to create a prayer box is a perfect exercise to go deeper within and figure out what you are wanting to happen on your journey. This is also a perfect way to spend time thinking and praying for yourself. Love yourself enough to be taking time to unravel wishes and prayers that are just waiting to be answered.

Not all of my prayers came true. But usually the few that didn't materialize were replaced with a better alternative or outcome. After three years or so, I had to go back to Tiffany's to buy a small gift for myself just to have another turquoise box. Oh, that prayer box was very special to me. What a comfort to hold something in my hand during uncertain times, faced with new places and friends. Something I could count on when I needed it the most.

What you need to make your prayer box:

- A small to medium-sized box. Get creative. Buy something pretty that will make your soul sing.

- Paper and pen (I suggest you handwrite your requests out instead of typing them. It's a more authentic touch).
- Tissue paper—to separate prayers 'still out for jury' and for answered ones on the bottom.

2. A special necklace

Okay, so you're not a Catholic. Neither am I. But I loved those beloved saints. I have read books on them, studied their lives and found much fascination in how they devoted their lives to creating a more loving, peaceful world without ever thinking of their needs first. Yes, you might have guessed now what my special necklace is. I wear a combination of saints around my neck: the miraculous medal, St Rita, and St Benedict. I keep them next to my bed. I hand them out as gifts. I wear them when I travel. I was once asked by my brother, "Do you believe those give you power? Are you hoping they save you?"

"No," I answered. "But it gives me comfort."

He seemed to understand that. That made sense to him. My brother might have been confused by the fact he knew we weren't Catholics, so why was his sister wearing a saints necklace?

Comfort. Security. And a go-to object that is attainable that I can hold and feel in my hand when my world might seem vulnerable or uncertain. I have had these necklaces off and on throughout the years. I can't tell you the simple joy of just holding an actual thing that can stay with me and provide a moment of relief from fear. Especially during my thirties after my divorce, I found much comfort in keeping this necklace on and distributing several to friends and some homeless folks who just might be on a corner and looking forlorn. You never know, that one tangible item might have begun a seed of hope to change their life.

Isn't that what we all want? Hope? A little something to keep us going? If you are opposed to the saints, try something special to your heart and wear it on a long dog-tag-like chain that is easy to take on and off.

I gave a saint necklace once to a new friend of mine who I did not know was an atheist. She was so touched I gave her something tangible to hold with special meaning to me. As she walked off, she said, "I shall wear it always." I loved that. See? Everyone needs something tangible to hold onto... My new friend was over the 80-years-old bracket and a neurophysicist to boot. I have been touched by her kindness in my life as well.

What you need:

- A long chain (think like a dog-tag chain) 17 inches or longer
- A special memento that you can wear on your chain that has special meaning to your heart

You never know when you might just need instant comfort at the bottom of your fingertips. You will be happy you have that something special with you...always.

3. An inspirational book

Sorry, techie lovers. I am not talking about e-books or Kindle or Nook. This one has to be a hard bound or, at least, a paperback version that is real and you can feel it in your hands. Your Soul Kit needs three tangible items and the third is no exception to the rule. What is my inspirational book?

The Bible.

Yep. Pretty simple. It's gone with me everywhere. There is a reason why the Gideons are distributing the most popular book ever in the world of reading to every hotel room on the planet. They know the great secret of grace and comfort it offers to all. This is not exclusive, like some crazy religious fanatics would have you thinking. This is an inclusive book for all. Sixty authors come together to tell their story of the beginning of time, the wars and scary dark places that have wrecked nations, and stories of love and grace. These are examples that you can read over and over. I have sat on the floor on a dark bathroom furry rug by candlelight meditating with my hands on the Bible. Much comfort came from seeking this immediate contact from a tangible book that inspires me. I have it with me still by my bed in a white wicker basket sitting on top of another pile of books.

If you are opposed to the Bible for whatever reason, choose another book that holds a dear meaning to your heart. Make sure it is one with the language of love and grace. Make sure it's one that helps heal your scary moments with positive quotes that can help you get through the darkest hour to see the sun rise again tomorrow.

What you need:

- A book—hardcover or paperback will work.
- Make sure it's an inspirational read.

An e-book is off the list. It must be a tangible object you can feel when you need comfort. This is an awesome thing to have at your fingertips.

Just like 'the road less travelled,' M. Scott Peck revealed in his groundbreaking, awe-inspiring self-help book in 1982 that "Life is difficult." So make sure you have your own *Soul Kit* to take with you. Those three little items just might help you weather your next storm with shock absorbers.

Act as if what you do makes a difference. It does.
~ William James

Chapter 36

Tidy the Soul

Okay. Let's get down to basics. Most of us know these things. But sometimes it's good to have a reminder. Especially with hit shows like *Hoarder* on cable and everyone tuning in to see what's behind the closed doors of someone else's home.

What does your home look like on the inside? Are you proud of your home? Or is it in a constant state of clutter where you feel a little overwhelmed when you look in the corners?

A few years ago, I attended a seminar with another friend on the value of 'cleaning out your closet' to allow for new growth and excitement. I remember thinking that this sounded rather basic and cliché. Who hasn't heard this one? But after an hour of listening to this mini-guru on closet cleaning and spiritual rewards, I found myself understanding a little bit more of why this is important. You know, sort of similar to 'closing one door and another one will open.' However, according to her, this was not going to happen if you had hoards of material things, belongings shoved in the closets and in drawers in your home.

"Go home and clean out that closet," she instructed the class. Well, okay then. I did just that. Who would have guessed just how right she was! It seemed the more I cleaned and organized my things, the better I felt on the inside. I do believe there was even more to what she was explaining. I didn't experience some incredible miracle of something brand new materializing. I did, however, find myself a little lighter in my step and happier with myself because of taking her advice.

Don't worry and don't go thinking I was one of those hoarder types. No. I just liked to keep things and keep them in boxes and keep them with me in each chapter of change. Well, it doesn't take a rocket scientist to figure out that unloading unneeded things in our closet can cure some of what may be nagging at us on the inside.

But how many of us keep our lives in tip-top shape? I have a confession to make. Mine always happens to be my car. It's sometimes overwhelmed with little things from the week before. I need to apply these rules to this part of my life, too.

Thomas Moore, the author of *Care of the Soul*, urges us to do the same thing. By taking care of our environment and our things, we in turn are nourishing our souls by caring for the immediate life we experience every day.

You might find out after getting your little world organized, you won't be wanting a vacation as much when you start tidying your soul.

My mom called me one day to share something on happiness she had just heard on a talk show: *"Do just one thing to be happy. Just one thing."* My mom told me about this one day. She asked me if I wanted to know what the one thing was. Well, yes! Do spill the beans on this happiness piece that can brighten my day, Mom.

Make your bed every day and you will be happy.

Hmm. I must admit I was a bit let down by this revelation. I was expecting something grand—huge, earth-shattering news that would really motivate me. Well, always one to test a theory, I began, without fail, making my bed every morning before I took my son to school—and his, too. I took it a step further by making sure the dishes and kitchen were tidied, too.

Of course, as you might expect, dear reader, I found myself smiling more and less stressed when I walked in the door after a long day. I could go into my room and plop down on my gloriously made bed. I might even kick up my heels and gaze out my window for a bit and notice the beauty of the trees, then read a few pages from my favorite book. My bedroom has now become my sanctuary of escape. When I walk in, I see pale teals and blues and frilly happy pillows in a neat row after I have exited the hustle and bustle of life. I find moments of peace from my actions of 'tidying the soul.' I have applied these simple fundamentals to my daily routine and been rewarded for my actions.

So make sure you take care of your belongings. Your life and your décor at home. Unclutter your space and take time to keep things tidy.

Take Care of Your Diet and Your Health

Now that we have tidied our home and our soul is feeling a bit lighter, it's time to look into the mirror and assess what we see. How is your health? Yes, a mirror. You can pretty much gauge how healthy you are by looking at yourself and what you see. Is your skin ashen? Are there bags under your eyes? Does your skin look dry? Are you feeling the 'tire effect' in the mid-section on your mid-life journey?

In simple laymen's terms:

- Are you overweight?
- Are you eating healthy foods?
- Are you getting enough sleep?
- Do you drink enough water each day?
- Are you working out regularly? Do you exercise or at least go for walks? Or are you one of those bon-bon eaters living moment to moment on your technology gadgets, furiously eating empty calories lacking nutrients and still in starvation mode?

It can happen to the best of us. I mentioned in my book, *Middle Age Beauty*, that I gained weight when I became engaged to my husband. Too much celebrating over love, social drinking and heavy foods. Pizza and red wine with my girlfriends; we were having fun eating and drinking and living the good life. The good life can add up to bad health, and ugly big-girl pants. So don't let this become you.

And what is the result of our health and diet being out of whack or alignment? Self-loathing

- The inner critic runs amuck.
- Shame fills our daily walk.
- We lose our sparkle.
- We lose precious extra years to our life by living an unhealthy life today.

Well, don't worry! It's not too late to get on the health bandwagon. From gluten free, to Paleo, to Zone, to vegan, to counting calories, to juicing vegetables and fruits, there are lots of fabulous options out there to help you get back in sync with yourself/soul and body.

Eat healthy, get fit and the result will be that you will feel happier. It's just the natural outcome of taking care of our souls. Our soul is encased in our body. So make sure you aren't shying away from the mirrors in your home or being okay with increasing your pant size.

Here are a couple of fabulous documentaries that will inspire you to align your health/body and soul:

- *Fat, Sick and Nearly Dead*
- *Hungry for Change*

When I first watched Joe Cross's documentary, *Fat, Sick and Nearly Dead*, I was so impressed with all of the facts and science included on why juicing is one of the most powerful tools for 'rebooting' your body, as he has coined the phrase. If you can't figure out why people are juicing and you think it's bonkers, go online and watch his documentary *free*. That's right, it's free. Joe has dedicated his life to educating not just you and me, but the world on why this is the ticket to staying happy and healthier. Find him on Twitter or Facebook. I recommend following his Facebook page.

Hungry for Change is a documentary that interviews world-famous nutritionists and experts on why obesity is on the rise and how we can actively reverse this cycle. They examine the food pyramid and discuss why our bodies like to store sugar immediately into fat when we eat it (think caveman days here). This is an excellent educational piece with inspiring stories that can help you get on your way. Check out their Facebook page, too. I follow Joe Cross's and Hungry for Change for daily reminders and inspiration.

One of the first and foremost things we can do to actively change and improve our moods is manage what we eat. Like I said before in *Middle Age Beauty*,

Choose you before you choose your food.

Mother Nature Is Calling

Okay, you technology-lovers out there who read Forbes Technology page online and keep yourself glued to your smart-phone, tablet, computer or flat screen:

Turn them off and go outside and connect with Mother Nature. My nature walks and little peaceful getaways to the country, park or to the beach are my chance to become reflective and tap into myself. When the world of lights and gadgets is turned off, we are left with a little more time to check in with our world. So take a step back from those fabulous apps. Stop playing those games so much and schedule mini-nature breaks. Nothing soothes the soul more than a nice supply of healthy oxygen to our bloodstream. So breathe an ocean breeze. Take long, meaningful walks under the shaded trees in Central Park (always be safe first!) and get in touch with fresh air and peace.

So let's do the round-up time. What three little things are you going to make sure you are doing to add a bit of extra bliss into your schedule?

1. Tidy your soul—make your bed!
2. Make your health and diet a priority.
3. Make time for Mother Nature (this absolutely includes exercising).

Your exercise for the week: Clean one closet. Go for a nature hike and watch a health food documentary to inspire your inner soul to reach up and help redesign a healthier and better you. It's fun to keep your body in shape. And it's fun to make a day out of cleaning your closets. You will even enjoy a documentary on why you should be eating more fruits and vegetables. So get with it and *tidy your soul* with these simple tips that can help add some verve and enthusiasm to your weekly schedule.

Anyone who truly loves God, travels securely.
~ Saint Teresa of Avila

Chapter 37

The Safety Net for the Soul

During my divorce at the beginning of the millennium I was uncertain of my future and where my life was headed. Those who divorce don't ever expect to divorce and that wasn't part of my original path. As life unfolded, though, that ended up being part of my story.

I have discussed this period of my life earlier in the book and there is a reason why it comes up the most. It was by far the most challenging and scary part of my journey.

This is what I thought my life would look like:

- Fun times
- Career driven
- Married with babies

I never thought:

- Divorced
- Single mother
- Must now come up with a new career

That just didn't seem to fit my ideas as a bright and bubbly 18-year-old headed out on the path of her dreams and desires.

Sometimes life takes us down new paths that are our choices. Our choices change us and we create a new reality. And then sometimes, new circumstances emerge, forcing us to change a reality we never wanted to change. Did you get that? I hope you did. Life can be complicated. Life isn't just a fairy tale after all. And even though Audrey Hepburn—my favorite Icon ever—still believed in fairy tales, the truth in life can be a much more bitter pill to swallow. (I do agree, though. I do think that it is worth believing in those wonderful fairy tales. Sometimes that is all that keeps us going.)

So. I don't want to be 'Woe is me' here, but you get the picture. A 32-year-old divorced, single mom living in the suburbs of San Diego with a feeling of dread hanging over her head. Is that okay to admit? Just admit the truth? That most dreaded of dreaded feelings is just...*dread*.

What to do? Where to go? I ask you? I tell you? Do you know? This is where you have to get creative, become soulful, and create and find a space where you can soothe those inner demons that threaten to take you down the road of the Pity Party. Yes!

Silence that voice that threatens to tell you:

You are Nothing! Who do you think you are to think you are Something?

Don't listen to the small inner critic. You know, that little voice that continues to believe and want smaller things for you in your life because that seems like the easier route.

Before I moved to San Diego, I had discovered in Los Angeles that if I visited certain places during scary and uncertain times, my soul felt a reprieve from that inner mean voice. I could escape it. I could find...yes, a 'Safety Net for My Soul.'

When I lived in Los Angeles, I had plenty of spots. I had them in treasure troves because I guess I really needed them up there. I would wander down to Malibu on the weekends and sit next to the ragged rocks standing gracefully next to the bluff of the California coastline. I would sit there on my towel and look out over the horizon. I could sit there for a few hours alone. It was so peaceful and relaxing. One time a naked man from the topless beach nearby invaded my view. He kept prancing around in front of my horizon, but I never looked at him. I could only see the ocean meeting the great blue sky off in the distance. This naked weirdo was not going to ruin my happy place. I could be stubborn like that. Yes.

Another spot was of course a beautiful Catholic cathedral just a hop, skip and a jump from Hollywood Studios. I would wander through the big open wooden doors, sprinkle holy water on my face, and then wish for the best. I would kneel in silence on the folded-down piece that allowed me to get close to God and then I would pray. I could sit there for an hour or so, and anything uneasy or scary bothering my soul would just lift up into the air and be carried away by the grace and the beauty of my surroundings.

Another spot was a bookstore in Studio City just off of Tujunga. It was known as 'the smallest bookstore in the world.' Great name. Great place. I found out recently that it went out of business. My heart sank at that.

Well, let me speed you up to the part of my journey where I found myself divorced and looking at a plateau off the side of an apartment in Carmel Valley. I hadn't prepared for that kind of change. And I thought that marriage and babies would carry me through the last chapter of my life (naiveté strikes the best of us when we are young).

So where was my Safety Net there? Yes, I had a church I went to…that counted. Yes, I found the beach there, too. But my favorite spot ended up being this little Catholic shop on Mira Mesa Boulevard. The owner's name was Rick, I think. He was so lovely. I found it when I went looking to buy some saint medals. I never knew that first day, that place would be my comfort and joy over the next few years.

When you walked through the door, a bell above your head, placed on the door, would ring. Then a surge of choir singers playing on a CD for sale would serenade and welcome you, too. The aisles of books, saints, relics, clocks, ceramic doves and wooden rosary boxes just looked so lovely and sweet to me. I would check them each out and then make my way to the back of the store where Rick would always be.

"Hi, Machel."

"Hi, Rick. How are you today?"

"As good as can be expected. I hope for the best. I haven't gotten in those miracle medals you were looking for last time. My shipment from Italy hasn't arrived yet."

"That's okay. I can look for something else..."

"Don't forget to have a cookie on the table and some coffee."

"Thanks, Rick."

I hate to say one word negative about my happy spot, but the coffee was rather strong and the cookies rather boring. But I always had one of each like it was the best thing I had ever eaten. At that moment it was because I was in my 'Safety Net for My Soul' place. I felt good there. Life was safe. And I could find peace and quiet there whenever it was open. I started a habit of buying long chains with saint medals and giving them out to my friends. I always bought a few. I felt like I was sharing part of my soul with them. To this day, I still keep these saints next to me. And, no, I was not raised Catholic. I just happened to love those saints and all their stories of what they did to attain peace and to be closer to God.

I think when it comes down to it, that is what we all want. Just a little peace and quiet. A place to call our own and a feeling that we are loved.

I even took my parents to this shop one time when they came out to visit me. I remember looking at my dad's expression. He was wondering, "What happened to the beach and why have you brought me to a Catholic shop? I was raised Baptist!"

But once he met Rick, had a cookie and a cup of coffee, my dad never poked fun at me about my love for this Catholic shop. I think he loved it, too.

Tears fill my eyes as I tell you now that the shop is gone. I do not know where Rick and his family went. I am sure he is fine.

But his business closed one day when I was away for too long of a stretch and I never found out what happened.

Where is my place now? I guess I could say home. I have found it finally at Home. I do sometimes wander to the sands of the beach and the windy waves of the ocean for soothing therapy to connect me to Mother Nature. I still do love a good bookstore and a coffee shop. I have a certain love for a yogurt shop that makes almond-milk ice cream. I can order it, and feel instantly happy. I am peaceful there.

So, dear reader, if you don't have your Safety Net for the Soul type place yet, get busy and look for one! It could be right under your nose. It's so wonderful to have a certain spot that is outside our normal routine that can soothe our soul and bring us a moment of joy. One more quick example would be my husband's place. He loves to visit pet stores in our area and buy our animals treats. I always watch Robin's face as it lights up with moments of joy as he finds new toys for our pets and yummy treats to spoil them with at home.

Safety Net for the Soul

(A place outside your normal routine that can bring joy or bliss by just visiting this place)

Examples:

- A hiking trail
- A coffee shop
- A church
- A store that brings you joy when you shop there (I am not talking about Nordstrom!)
- A green meadow in a field near where you live
- The park in your neighborhood
- A grand tree that you may love to sit underneath
- The beach

In life, there will come a time when you will seek a place away from your routine that can add a moment of grace to your schedule. Go deep within and search for what makes you happy and find a spot near your home that can add that safety net you may be missing out on each week. Get busy and find the spot your soul needs when life is crazy.

Know thyself. Then you shall know the universe and God.
~ Pythagoras

Chapter 38

Interview—with You, Dear Reader. Unlock Your Goals and Dreams

Now as we come to the end of the book, I am going to share the most important interview with you—YOURS!

What is it that you want out of this life? Do you have a list? A dream? A thought or a whimsical notion? I hope you take this time to sit in your quiet spot with your pen or pencil and take time to write inside this book. Fill out your dreams. Your aspirations. Tell me your deepest desires! I want you to feel like the Rock Star you are. I want you to believe in your dreams. Yes, this life can be a struggle. You will have ups and downs. There is no easy road. There is no way out of the struggle. It happens to all of us. Even to those who you think have it all. It is up to us to have our souls armed and ready to live this life with a bright and bold smile. Are you ready to do some internal work? Are you ready to dig out of your mind your hopes and dreams…at the age of 25 or the age of 85? Life is a beautiful stage for us to fill with our own props, characters and stories. Make sure you are telling the story you want to tell. After all, this is your life. You can be the dream you want to become.

Your Interview

Are you happy with your current circumstances in your life right now? If there is anything you can change, what would it be?

Your answer:

Do you have a bold and beautiful dream you have always wanted to happen? What is it? Write it down now. Now write a paragraph on what it would feel like if you could make this dream happen. What actions or steps could you create to begin this process?

Your answer:

Do you have a resentment or grievance with someone or something from your past? If so, write it down. (You can just add initials if writing a name is too painful.) Now what would you say to this person? Write that out now.

Your answer:

Now imagine filling your heart with love and compassion for this person who you feel has hurt you. Make amends by filling your mind with the power of love and thoughts of peace. Imagine making peace with them even if you know this will never happen. Write what that would feel like now.

Your answer:

What do you like about yourself? Write out a list now of your best attributes. Add a little story on something you did that made you feel proud. Now write down one more thing that you would like to do to emulate this feeling.

Your answer:

Do you have a faith system? What is it? If not, do you think that adding something more to believe in than just yourself could add comfort to your soul? What would it feel like to know there is a higher power that is always loving you and watching out for you?

Your answer:

Do you know what little things you can do right now that can add happiness to your daily routine? Write those out now.

Your answer:

Can you imagine yourself feeling happy every day? What would that feel like when you wake up? Write that now. Okay, now take the time to think for a moment what that would be like and add, in your mind: "I can be this person. I can add joy to my life with little moments of bliss by discovering what I love inside. I can do internal work to make my life more fun and pleasant by wanting to know who I am on the inside." Now write down three things you will do each week to actively seek happiness in your life.

Your answer:

What would it feel and look like if you were more joyful each day by taking action and making that happen?

Your answer:

I hope this interview with yourself helped to reveal something new and exciting. I hope you make more time for YOU and get busy loving yourself more each day. This was the most important interview of the book. YOURS. I wish I could read your words and see what you revealed. I am sure they are honest words from your heart. I am sure they reveal to you your stronger self. I am sure of YOU.

Prayer is not asking. It is a longing of the soul. It is a daily admission of one's weakness. It is better in prayer to have a heart without words than words without a heart.

~ Mahatma Gandhi

Chapter 39

Epilogue

Well, dearest reader, I am sorry to say goodbye right now. I feel as if we have taken a journey together. I feel like together we have gotten to know each other better by sharing what our thoughts and dreams are. I cannot hear what yours are, but I can imagine them as I write this. I think we are all connected by our wishes and dreams. We were all children at one time gazing up at the stars and dreaming big dreams and believing in them. We have similar wants and needs. Life can be unexpected, scary and sad. But don't let your obstacles defeat you. You can get to know and love yourself more by making an effort to go within. You are worth the journey, aren't you?

So put down your tablets, and those smartphones. Stop surfing the web and go within. Question your thinking, your likes, and discover who and what makes you tick. Learn to love those who are surrounding your path, too. Honor their stories. Share yours. Be vulnerable. Love. Pray more. Show compassion. Be strong. Live. This life is such a beautiful journey. Don't be dismayed by the pain. Instead fight to win one more day of serenity for your soul. Fight to be that person who smiles a real smile from within. There is no reason to pretend, my friend. Life is too beautiful to numb ourselves to the glory of its journey. You deserve to live loud, love more, and share more of your soul. Your soul is waiting to be discovered. Uncover it, and tap into your natural right to be happy.

I wish you well. Please think big and happy thoughts. Shoot for those fondest dreams. Have hopes for tomorrow. Anything is possible when you believe. I thank you for taking time to share your story with me inside my book. I hope this helps you discover your own ways to your inner happiness on your journey.

Also, remember to share your love with others. Don't under-estimate the power of love. Thank you! I am grateful for you. I wish you well on your journey. And remember to hold on to one more day. Something new and wonderful could be just around the corner.

Best wishes with love,

~ Machel (*Mimi* for short)

*If you are suffering from depression, please seek help immedi-ately and reach out to those you love.

Suicide Hotlines
US

1 (800) 273-8255 **National Suicide Prevention Lifeline**
Hours: 24 hours, 7 days a week
Languages: English, Spanish
Website: www.suicidepreventionlifeline.org

International Suicide Prevention
ISAP
International Association for Suicide Prevention
http://www.iasp.info/resources/Crisis_Centres/Europe/
(individual listed phone numbers are there for each country)